ACKNOWLEDGEMENTS

Dr Fredric Brandt would like to thank:
My patients, who through the years have inspired my creativity;
my staff in Miami and New York; Patricia Reynoso for adding style to
my words; my personal assistant Maggie, who is brilliant at keeping my
life in order; my head nurse Susie Salviejo; Dr Andres Boker, research
scientist extraordinaire; my agent, Lisa Queen and my editor Claire Wachtel,
for their enormous patience; Nada Lantz at Lantz-a-Lot for her endless
enthusiasm; Jackie Tractenberg and Dana Tuchman at Tractenberg & Co.;
our volunteers, Maija Arbolino, Brenda Segel, Linda Asch and Andrea
Cantor, who generously submitted their faces for everyone to see; our
photographer, Sonja Pacho, and her talented team: Miok (hairstyling),
Gail Goodman (make-up), Gina Appleby (styling) and Ronald Cadiz. Also,
Bobbi Queen, Joy Behar and my beautiful golden retriever, Sparky.
Finally, the late Dr Harvey Blank, former chairman of the department
of dermatology at the University of Miami, whose vast knowledge
continues to inspire me in the daily practice of dermatology.

Patricia Reynoso would like to thank:
Dr Brandt, for always returning my phone calls; my husband,
Euclide, for his endless reserves of patience and encouragement;
my sister, for being my cheerleader; my friends and colleagues at
W, Jane Larkworthy and Dahlia Devkota, for generously lending
me out and my twins, Brandon and Grace, whose flawless skin
is so inspiring.

CONTACT DETAILS

New York office:
317 East 34th Street
6th Floor
New York
NY 10016
USA
tel (00 1) 212 889 7096

email: DERMBRANDT@aol.com
website: www.drbrandtskincare.com

Miami office:
4425 Pont de Leon Blvd
Suite 200
Coral Gables
FL 33146
USA
tel (00 1) 305 443 6606

INTRODUCTION

I don't think I could have picked a more exciting time to be a cosmetic dermatologist. My twenty years in practice have exposed me to a multitude of patients seeking answers to the same burning question: how can we slow down this speeding train called the ageing process? Clearly, there's no bringing that train to a halt – at least not in this era – but if there's one point that I try to convey to the men and women who sit in my chair, it's that there's never been a better time to seek a little rejuvenation.

The last two decades have been incredible in terms of learning about what damages and prematurely ages the skin, and better yet, realising how this damage can be prevented, and even repaired. Before then, little was said about the ageing role of sun exposure, smoking, pollution, deficient nutrition and even stress. We thought that lines and wrinkles were an unavoidable rite of passage and that a mediocre complexion could never be more than just that. Persistent acne was tolerated, while sun spots were often blamed on eating too much liver – I kid you not! At best, a visit to the dermatologist was reserved for an itchy rash or an annoying wart. Finally, when it came to at-home skin care, the majority reached for a bar of soap and perhaps slathered on cold cream if they were feeling adventurous.

Oh, how times have changed! Today we know that a suntan should come from a bottle of self-tanning lotion and that your dermatologist's number is worthy of a place in your speed-dial. Similarly, celebrating your God-given looks is admirable, but that doesn't make it wrong to want to improve upon them. On a related note, our narrow definition of beauty has finally burst open enough so that a Barbie doll's long, blonde hair and blue eyes aren't the only standard to strive for. We've seen this in Hollywood, too. At the 2002 Academy Awards, best actress winner Halle Berry was just as breathtaking on the podium as was Julia Roberts the year before.

One cannot discuss the effects of ageing without bringing up the 'baby boomer' population. On estimate, 35% of the UK's population was born between 1946 and 1964, forming a massive group of people prepared to fight their way into prolonged youthfulness. Today, the oldest baby boomers are entering their mid-50s and the youngest are already in their late 30s, meaning that there is probably no end in sight to this obsession with the ageing process. My patients are in this very age group and if there's one sentiment that I hear over and over again, it's that while they understand they have to age, they plan to do it their way. Staying youthful and beautiful just for the sake of staying young and beautiful is no longer enough. Beauty equates with power and control and for the baby boomers, that in itself is more valuable than anything else. To quote one of my good patients, 'I thought I could age gracefully, but nah, that's out the window now!'

The influx of information and innovation that has hit the skin care market, both in products and in cosmetic procedures performed at a dermatologist's office, has had an immense impact on how we treat the ageing process. The advent of 'cosmeceuticals', an entirely new genre of skin care products that are known to deliver a biological action on the skin yet are sold over the counter, is a prime example of this. A host of ingredients are in this category, and they include retinol, alpha and beta hydroxy acids, and antioxidants – with many others joining this prestigious group on a constant basis. Prescription skin medications, such as *Retin-A*, are also a great option for a significant number of people.

The other half of the equation is reflected in the leaps and bounds happening in the dermatologist's office. It seems hard to imagine a time when a facelift was considered to be the best solution for turning back the clock. In reality this perception couldn't have been farther from the truth. When the facelift was finally performed, the result was old skin that still looked old except it was now pulled back – not exactly the picture of youthfulness.

Plastic surgery remains a viable option for a lot of people, but it's definitely not the universal solution that it was once considered to be. We now know that a facelift only addresses a portion of the ageing process that is affecting your appearance. Issues like deep lines on the forehead and sides of the mouth, and skin that has lost its youthful glow remain stubbornly intact – even after the best surgery with the best plastic surgeon in town. The radiant fullness of the face is, in my opinion, one of the most important signs of youth, and plastic surgery will definitely not bring that back. Clearly, the key to erasing a few years off the face will not be found in the plastic surgeon's office.

This is where superior at-home skin care and dermatological procedures like acid peels, filler injections, non-burning lasers and *Botox* come into play. Together they allow you to control how you look, regardless of your chronological age. The bottom line is: take care of your skin in small ways today and you might never need to go under the knife tomorrow.

Even those who have already taken the leap into plastic surgery will benefit from taking charge of their skin. Whatever led them to the plastic surgeon in the first place will send them back there if they don't keep up the good work at home. I see many patients who have had facial plastic surgery and I count them among my best clients. One female patient even told me that her hairstylist had accused her of having had a second facelift – he simply couldn't believe how rested and rejuvenated she seemed. When he demanded to know her secret, she told him that she'd been tinkering with *Botox*.

We cannot deny that attractiveness is still a very powerful tool. Like it or not, others judge us by our appearance. I'll even venture to say that there might never be a time when looks don't matter. But if there's one message I want to convey it's that beauty lies in the eye of the beholder – yours. Take advantage of the vast array of information and technology that you're lucky to have at your disposal and bring your very best face forward.

NOTE TO READER

This book is designed to provide information about the various remedies for ageing that are presently available, to help you become a more informed consumer of these medical and health services. It is not intended to be complete or exhaustive, but is based solely on the professional opinions of Dr Fredric Brandt, whose opinions may not reflect every doctor's viewpoint. Before you undergo any cosmetic procedure, it is wise to first have an in-depth consultation with your health care provider. The author and the publisher expressly disclaim responsibility for any adverse effects arising from the use or application of the information contained herein.

PART ONE

COVERING THE BASICS

CHAPTER ONE
IN THE BEGINNING

Answer me this: what is the largest organ in the body that regulates body temperature, protects us from dehydration and injury and can feel many sensations, including pain, heat and cold? Need another clue? Its flawless, radiant appearance can make the difference between a good day and a fantastic day. Funny, isn't it, how the answer suddenly seems so clear?

The condition of the skin is a national obsession and understandably so. Think back to the great beauties of our time (Grace Kelly, Marilyn Monroe and Elizabeth Taylor circa *Cat on a Hot Tin Roof* spring to mind) and while they may have differed in colouring, hairstyles, physique and fashion sense, they all shared a common trait. You guessed it – they all possessed complexions so awe inspiring that the heart aches just looking at their photographs. We have our share of celebrated beauties today, and once again the common denominator is their smooth complexion, even skin tone, full lips, radiant glow and utter lack of wrinkles. Beautiful skin is a valuable commodity and better yet, one that is within reach.

Aiming for beautiful skin is a worthy goal, and we will be discussing the many ways to achieve it, but I also want to emphasise that just like any other organ in the body, the skin needs to be protected and cared for. When you tend to your skin – by shielding it from the sun's damaging rays, eating nutrient-rich foods, sleeping adequately, using superior skin care products and entrusting its care to a dermatologist – it will reward you with an envy-inducing, healthy appearance.

···⟩ serves as an
environmental barrier

···⟩ protects us from water
loss and wounds

···⟩ uses specialised pigment
cells to protect us from the
sun's rays

···⟩ helps regulate body
temperature through
sweat glands

···⟩ is involved in the production
of vitamin D

THE LIVING SKIN

At first glance the skin seems pretty unremarkable, just a thin,
flesh-toned covering for the body. But if you could peek inside, the
sophisticated network within would amaze you. Generally speaking,
the skin is divided into two layers: the epidermis and the dermis.

EPIDERMIS

Whenever you study your skin or run your hands over it, you're
touching the top layer, known as the epidermis. The epidermis is
partially responsible for the skin's colour, texture and overall
appearance. It also helps the skin stay moisturised by retaining water
and acting as a barrier from the sun. Have you ever wondered how
we're able to live on land and swim in the sea? You can thank the
epidermis, for it is impermeable to water.

Topping the epidermis is the *stratum corneum*, and that is what we
see when we undergo our weekly sessions with the magnifying mirror.
This coating is made up of flattened dermal cells which lie on the
stratum corneum in a basketweave pattern. These cells were once
baby cells that, in a process called cell renewal, migrate to the top. In
healthy adults, this process happens over a fifteen to thirty day period,
and as we age, the process slows down considerably.

Deeper in the epidermis are the three other layers: the transitional
layer, the suprabasal layers and the basal layer. In some ways, all are
responsible for the overall health and beauty of the skin.

DERMIS

In the world of beauty, the dermis is a virtual treasure trove, especially since it is where our precious collagen and elastin fibres reside. In fact, almost 70% of the dermis is made up of collagen, with the remainder consisting of elastin, blood vessels, sebaceous glands, sweat glands, hair follicles and immune system cells. This layer of skin is also incredibly resilient and can absorb a great amount of pressure.

THE FATTY LAYER

Composed mostly of fat cells and elastin fibres, the fatty layer is the deepest layer of the skin and works to insulate us and shield our inner organs from harm. This layer varies in thickness depending on where it is on our skin. Not surprisingly, it's pretty thick on our abdominal areas, whilst almost nonexistent on the eyelids. On the other parts of the body, it's also where the dreaded condition of cellulite makes its appearance.

But more importantly, let's discuss collagen and the role that it plays in the way your skin looks and behaves.

THE COLLAGEN CONNECTION

When your collagen is plentiful and healthy you will know it by what you see in the mirror. Think of collagen as your skin's mattress, and elastin as the coils that hold it together. Like everything else related to the ageing process, our collagen is at its most abundant during the early childhood years and anyone who has admired a toddler's velvety skin can attest to that. Collagen production slows down in puberty, levels off in your 20s and 30s and – you guessed it – grinds to a halt in later years.

The beauty world is obsessed with keeping collagen safe and sound, and considering what a fundamental role it plays in the maintenance of beautiful skin, this obsession is totally warranted. Perhaps more importantly, collagen helps to heal wounds and scars. Many creams claim to protect it, repair it and regenerate it, but there is scant evidence that any of them actually deliver these promises. (The only exception is the vitamin A derivative tretinoin, which studies show to have a positive effect on collagen.) Years ago, when the anti-ageing skin care market was in its infancy, there was an onslaught on 'collagen creams' that claimed to boost natural collagen. Most people lost faith in them when they realised that the collagen molecule contained in these creams – which was derived from cattle – was too large to penetrate to the skin's barrier. In other words, try, try again.

The fibroblast skin cells produce collagen and it is the degeneration of collagen, both through excessive exposure to the sun as well as extreme environmental conditions, that eventually leads to wrinkles and sagging skin. Once collagen is destroyed it is very difficult to reproduce. Some of the latest non-surgical cosmetic procedures, like collagen injections, help repair the harm, but nothing will ever bring it back to its virgin state.

ELASTIN

Known as collagen's partner in crime, elastin is another connective tissue found in the dermis. These stretchy fibres allow the skin to snap back into place. Over time, and with repeated sun exposure, the elastin breaks down into small fragments. There is no remedy for the destruction of elastin. When it's gone, it's pretty much gone.

OUR SKIN CELLS

- **Keratinocytes** The most abundant cell in the epidermis, these cells provide some of the rigidity of the outer layers of skin.
- **Fibroblasts** The king of all cells, fibroblasts produce collagen.
- **Melanocytes** Found in the epidermis, these cells produce the pigment melanin. As you're probably aware, melanin absorbs the harmful ultraviolet light produced by the sun and protects the skin's DNA from radiation damage. This pigment-producing cell also produces what is known as a tan, which sounds desirable, until you realise that a tan is simply the body's response to injury from ultraviolet radiation.
- **Langerhans** These cells are involved in the immune function of the skin.

FITZPATRICK SKIN TYPES

Developed by Professor Thomas Fitzpatrick, MD, PhD, as a classification system based on skin pigment to calculate sunlight burning, this system is commonly used as a guide for procedures that will affect pigmentation.

TYPE I
Extremely fair skin, red or blond hair, blue or green eyes
Always burns, never tans

TYPE II
Fair skin, sandy to brown hair, green or brown eyes
Usually burns, difficult to tan

TYPE III
Medium skin, brown hair, brown eyes
Sometimes burns, often tans

TYPE IV
Olive skin, brown or black hair, dark brown or black eyes
Rarely burns, tans with ease

TYPE V
Dark brown skin, black hair, black eyes
Very rarely burns, tans very easily

TYPE VI
Black or dark brown skin and hair, black eyes
Never burns, tans very easily

SKIN TYPES

It's impossible to intelligently peruse a skin care counter without first understanding what type of skin you call as your own. The typical classifications of oily, normal, combination and dry are still used today, but the rules of what constitutes each skin type aren't as hard and fast as they used to be. Most people may start out as one skin type and as they age and their skin changes, may wind up being something else entirely.

IN HARM'S WAY

Considering how miraculous the skin is, it's shocking how easy it is to take it for granted and to subject it to harm. Here are the top five bad habits that stand between you having the best skin possible. I'll be discussing it in more detail in *Chapter Two: What Ages Us?* but it's so important that it bears repeating.

···▷ Not using sunblock: keep this little formula in your head. You plus the sun minus the sunblock equals lots and lots of wrinkles.
···▷ Picking at your face: have you ever taken a good look at what's lurking underneath your fingertips as you zoom in on your face? It's not pretty, and neither will your skin be when it's left scarred and infected.

→ Not sleeping: maybe it's the martyr in all of us that likes to brag about our amazing two hours of sleep, but do this often enough and you'll be left with the skin to show for it. Take my advice and catch a few zzzz's.

→ Stressing out: our busy lifestyles have a way of turning us into hyperventilating maniacs. Before you continue to blow your cool, stop and remember that this is the easiest way to lower your immunity, and in the process cause your skin to flare up.

→ Poor nutrition: in the quest for perfect physiques, we have forgotten that starving ourselves can deplete our skin of essential nutrients. Trust me, a steady diet of rice cakes and diet soda will do nothing to enhance your complexion, and lots to ruin it.

No matter what your desired end result, it's important to treat our skin respectfully and as best as we can. Believe me when I say that there's never been a better time to achieve these goals. In the following chapters I will discuss the many transformations that the skin undergoes. Some, like natural ageing, are going to happen no matter what our intentions, while a larger part of it does lie within our control. However, once you understand why your skin behaves and looks the way that it does, half the beauty battle is already won.

CHAPTER TWO
WHAT AGES US?

When, exactly, did it all start? Where did the carefree days of your youth disappear to, the ones when only that occasional blemish could ruin your day? It's sneaky, I know, and even potentially distressing, but there's no way to avoid the fact that ageing will happen to each and every one of us. If we can't avoid it, then we might as well understand it, because this will teach us that there is a lot that we can do to slow this process down.

There are two basic types of ageing: intrinsic (or chronological) ageing and extrinsic (or sun-induced) ageing. The first type, intrinsic, refers to the inevitable passage of time and the conditions that arise because of it. In the 1960s, scientists discovered that the root cause of ageing lay deep within our skin cells' DNA – which is why it's a good idea to glance at your parents to see what the future holds for you. Some of the conditions that come with intrinsic ageing, which I will be describing in further detail later in this chapter, will happen no matter how well-intentioned you are. The good news – and anyone who is devoted to reading beauty magazines has certainly heard this before – is that there is plenty that you can do to lessen the appearance of intrinsic ageing characteristics.

The second type of ageing is a more sinister one, if only because it falls within our control yet delivers the majority of the harm that we view as aged skin. Extrinsic ageing is caused by external factors such as smoking, excessive use of alcohol, poor nutrition and, of course, the big one: sun exposure. Because this process is not inevitable, it is often referred to as premature ageing. More than 80% of the characteristics of prematurely aged skin can be attributed to sun exposure. It's also important to note that incidences of skin cancer occur almost exclusively in photo-aged skin.

AGEING BY TIME

Signs include:

⤳ Dry skin: as the oil glands stop working as hard to keep your skin moist, the result is skin with pronounced dehydration.

⤳ Wrinkles: those little worker bees known as collagen and elastin start to lose their strength, leaving the skin with some wrinkling.

⤳ Loss of skin elasticity: the loss of collagen and elastin are largely to blame for the appearance of wrinkles, but a lot of dynamic expressions – in the form of smiling, frowning, and squinting – contribute as well.

⤳ Enlarged pores: they're the bane of our existence, and I hate to deliver the news that they're not going anywhere soon. Some people are predisposed to having enlarged pores and others are blessed with nonexistent pores, but in both cases the loss of the skin's underlying support system causes them to open up even more with age.

⤳ Broken capillaries: these fine red lines appear most frequently on the cheeks and nose, and they're due to the proliferation of many tiny broken capillaries.

⤳ Increased healing time: our healing time begins to increase once we reach our 30s, with epidermal regeneration taking twice as long in our 70s and 80s as it did in our earlier years. The result is not only a dulled complexion, but also a longer wound-healing process.

AGEING BY SUN

Signs include:

···⟩ Increased roughness: as the sun destroys the skin's collagen and elastin, the skin becomes rough and less elastic.

···⟩ Spots everywhere: constant exposure to the sun's ultraviolet rays makes our skin pigment act abnormally, resulting in a litany of spots throughout the face, upper chest and hands.

···⟩ Cross-hatched wrinkling: a plastic surgeon interested in documenting the environment's effect on the skin decided to study identical twins who had led different lifestyles. In one case the twin who had taken care to stay out of the sun had considerably less wrinkling throughout her face, especially on her cheeks and forehead.

DON'T LET THE SUN SHINE ON YOU

I like to think of myself as fairly easygoing – there's very little that irks me and much more that makes me laugh out loud. But if a patient wants to see me come undone, they'd know to visit me with suntanned skin. Actually, I should change that to the less seductive, yet more realistic label of 'damaged' skin. On a daily basis I treat patients who are calmly waiting their turn to improve their complexions. Yet they feign innocence when I ask about the telltale signs – usually dark spots coupled with a bronzed, crinkled skin – littering their face, arms, hands and, most commonly, their chest.

The excuses come fast: 'I was wearing the sun block that you gave me,' swears the male half of the bronzed couple from Peru. Others are more belligerent: 'I'm not going to stop living so that I can look good at eighty,' says the thirty-two-year-old blonde estate agent with the snazzy convertible and a love of sailing.

Our dangerous love affair with the sun began almost sixty years ago, when tanned complexions were a sure sign that one worked outdoors for a living. Eventually, that changed to being a badge of honour among the chic – a sign that one had the means to spend weeks on a yacht in the Riviera. So pervasive was this image that even Coco Chanel fell into its grasp, becoming the first designer to parade bronzed mannequins on her catwalks. If the message wasn't clear before, it certainly was now: tanned was the ideal – at any cost. Just ask the Ambre Solaire model. Didn't she seem to be having a ball?

Appearances, no matter how utterly convincing, can be deceiving. The simple fact is that a darkened tone is the skin's immediate reaction to the damage that has been inflicted upon it. 'Damage' is the operative word here, because it is this very damage that will, without a doubt, show up as premature ageing on your skin. In other words, the majority of wrinkles and other signs of ageing don't have to be there at all. For every cautious, sunblock-wearing patient that I treat, I see five others flaunting their hard-earned tans. Yet these are the same people who will ask me to 'do something' about the lines and spots on their faces and bodies.

This might be the twenty-first century, but perhaps a repeat lesson on what a tan really is, is in order now.

THE FULL SUNTAN STORY

Anytime that unprotected skin (for which read, naked and devoid of sunblock) is exposed to the sun, an insidious cycle of damage is initiated almost immediately. The two ultraviolet rays that are found in sunlight, UVB and UVA, deliver their blows in different ways. The first, UVB, is often called the 'burning' ray because of its power to do just that. Anyone who has ever dealt with painful sunburns can thank good old UVB. The other, the UVA ray, doesn't burn the skin, but due to its longer wavelengths it is able to reach deeper into the skin, down to the cellular level, where our DNA resides. Combined, the two activate the free radical damage that we now know is largely to blame for the majority of skin ageing, not to mention a host of other diseases, like skin cancer.

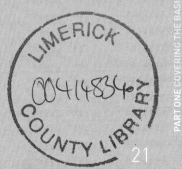

NOW, THE GOOD NEWS . . .

Living in Miami, a.k.a. the sunbathing capital of America, has provided me with ample examples, both in the office and outside it, of why we must limit our time spent in the sun. Notice that I don't say 'eliminate', because even I realise that people genuinely enjoy being in the sun. With that in mind, before dispensing sun protection advice, I first try to ascertain my patients' lifestyle and the reasons why they're in the sun. If, for example, someone tells me that they love to play golf, or that they regularly take their children to the playground, then we try to work around those outings. Believe it or not, staying away from the sun during peak burning hours of 11 a.m. to 4 p.m. makes a significant difference to how much you damage your skin. I'm proud to say that I've been able to transform many of my patients with just this guideline. After all, even I realise that life's too short to give up the things that truly fill us with joy.

   This next piece of advice is almost simplistic, but since I am constantly given a multitude of excuses as to why people are sunburned, I think it bears repeating. First, everyone needs to think of sunblock as being as vital as toothpaste and as indispensable as those pricey anti-ageing creams. No sunblock will offer you complete protection from the sun – you'd need to go outside immersed in a metal cage to accomplish that – but the options today are so wonderfully diverse that it's truly inexcusable not to use one. In fact, the current crop of sunscreens is light years ahead of its predecessors. Up until only a few years ago, traditional sunscreens only offered protection from UVB rays, partially because the non-burning UVA rays were incorrectly considered harmless. (Actually, one could get sunblocks that offered additional protection from UVA, but they were thick and opaque and very unpleasant to wear.) This development was a major turning point because finally there was a product with real sunscreening benefits minus any opaque residue! Today, pretty much every brand delivers this broad-spectrum protection.

Another great milestone in sun protection came via a process called 'micronisation' – which reduced the particle size of titanium and zinc oxide (the proven but unappealing sunblocks of the time). Before this breakthrough sunblocks were thick and opaque, and not cosmetically acceptable to the general public. They finally became available in a form that was practical for everyone – not just lifeguards for whom this thick stripe was a signature look.

THE LOWDOWN ON SPF

Unfortunately, the current system for calculating sun protection factor (SPF) in sunscreens is far from perfect. It was originally developed to measure only the sun's burning properties. For example, if someone were to sit outside without any protection and become burnt after a minute, then a sunscreen with an SPF 15 would allow them to stay in the sun for 15 minutes before burning. This calculation is effective for protecting against burning, but as we now know, you don't have to burn to get skin damage since the UVA rays don't burn.

You might have noticed that SPF is available in a vast range of numbers, starting as low as 4 and climbing as high as 45 (some European brands go as high as SPF 60). Some sun protection is better than no sun protection, but in my professional opinion, I would suggest that you stick to an SPF 30, which is known to absorb 97% of the sun's rays.

In some parts of Europe, there is an entirely different system for measuring sun protection. If you pick up a sunscreen on holiday, you might notice that printed on the bottle is an IPD number, or Immediate Pigment Darkening. There's been a lot of controversy over how to properly measure UVA rays; but no matter how this is determined, it's important for the market to come to an agreement on how to achieve this. Currently, whenever you buy an American sunblock, there is nothing that tells you how much UVA protection you are receiving. For now, look for sunblocks containing Parsol 1789, zinc oxide and titanium dioxide.

DAILY DOSES

If you're anything like the majority of my patients, you're probably thinking that you can skip right over my lectures on the sun since you're one of the smart ones; sunblock is the first item you pack when going on holiday or taking a long weekend away. While this sort of foresight is a step in the right direction, it falls short of the type of protection that is ideal. You see, the sun is out *all the time*, not just when you're on a beach in the Caribbean. It's out when you're driving to the office, walking along the pavement or even dining indoors at your favourite restaurant. Yes, I said indoors. UVA rays are able to penetrate through glass, so without adequate sun protection, you are at risk for some damage. Even in the dead of winter, you should make an effort to protect yourself. If not, over time, this accumulated damage will greet you in the mirror via a leathery complexion, those aforementioned sun spots and an abundance of lines throughout – particularly the deep ones in a cross-hatched pattern on the cheeks. Just think of the wrinkled neighbour in the Cameron Diaz movie *There's Something About Mary* to see exactly what you don't want to look like. Why wait until your skin is damaged beyond repair to start caring for it? Let's focus on preserving its beautiful integrity now.

CANCER CONCERNS

On a more ominous note, research has shown that skin cancer is the second most common cancer in the UK. About 1 in every 150-200 people in the UK will contract skin cancer in their lifetime; there are roughly 40,500 new cases each year, resulting in about 1,500 deaths. If you need another reason to avoid the sun, this is clearly the one.

Once you've honed in on your sunblock of choice, you have to make a commitment to using it properly. Before stepping outside, at least a teaspoon-sized portion should be applied to your bare face and given time to absorb. Those with very sensitive skin should seek a chemical-free option, such as one with zinc oxide or titanium dioxide, while those with acne-prone skin should use a gel-based formula. Also, consider your itinerary for the day and adjust your sun protection accordingly. Remember that sand and water deliver almost 100% reflection, so for that big outing make sure to have your new favourite product on hand and reapply often. Finally, reach for a hat and sunglasses before heading outdoors. Just remember that a hat on its own offers almost negligible protection, especially the flimsy straw hats so popular during the summer months. A dark canvas hat that doesn't let any light show through is your best bet. Also, remember that clothing offers a natural SPF and there's an innovative new product (available through online pharmacies in the UK) that allows you to add extra protection to your clothing simply by throwing it in the wash. Tinted windows block UVA and UVB rays, as do the white gloves that many of my Miami patients wear as they drive in the hot sun. Those are my favourite patients!

A trend emerged a few years ago on make-up, such as foundation, that came already loaded with sunscreen, and while I think it's a step in the right direction, I still insist that you use a traditional sunscreen. Why? Firstly, most make-ups include only a minute amount of sunscreen. Secondly, and perhaps most importantly, recent studies show that sunscreen in make-up virtually disappears a mere two hours after application, leaving you with only the assumption of protection. Honestly, I resent the false sense of security that they deliver. The bottom line is: always use a separate sunscreen.

You've probably heard that over 80% of sun damage is received before the age of 18 and judging by the many patients who have sat in my office and reminisced about having suntanning competitions when they were teenagers, I'm not surprised. I think this statistic is worth repeating, but I also hesitate to bring it up because some sun fanatics might translate it as an invitation to indulge in even more damage. The damage is already done, right? But please, let's remember that those were the days when baby oil was the tanning tool of choice and ignorance was bliss, and we now know that no excuse is good enough for voluntarily speeding the ageing process. Even after years of tanning, someone who becomes serious about sun protection can achieve a great improvement in his or her skin's condition. The body is amazingly efficient at fighting free radical damage, especially when it's given a helping hand. I hope that the message is clear: embrace a natural aesthetic. Your face – and your dermatologist – will thank you for it.

To talk solely about the sun and the tick-tocking of the clock doesn't paint the full ageing picture. Here are some other big contributors:

DEFICIENT NUTRITION

I'm a big believer in that if you take care of your body and your health, of course it's going to be reflected in your overall appearance. Vitamins and natural antioxidants found in food, such as the healing lycopene antioxidant that is so prevalent in tomatoes, help the skin stay healthy and functioning properly. It's important to also keep your body in good shape, as the natural consequence of too much fat in the form of clogged arteries won't allow enough blood to get to where it needs to go.

SMOKING

It's beyond me why anyone would still want to smoke after knowing how unhealthy it is for every organ in the body. Perhaps I can appeal to our vain side by stating that it can also do a destructive number on your skin.

Formally, there are varying opinions on the effects of smoking on the skin. Some studies have demonstrated that smoking doesn't harm the skin that drastically, while others dispute those claims. My personal and professional opinion is that smoking adversely affects the skin in many ways. In fact, I can spot a smoker's skin immediately, as it tends to develop a very sallow appearance. Smokers also get a lot more blackheads, because the pores are so dilated due to the decrease of collagen in the skin. Smokers also don't heal as quickly as non-smokers, a consideration that has prompted many plastic surgeons to refuse to operate on smokers.

SLEEPLESS NIGHTS

The next time you're tempted to trade a few hours of sleep for a few more hours at the office, remember that while you're snoozing, the body is recuperating. It is a known fact that while we sleep the body is working harder than ever to regenerate and unwind from the tensions of the day. While we sleep, our bodies secrete growth hormones that are responsible for restoring cells and building skin, hair and bone. Rob your body of enough sleep and you'll start to see the consequences in your red eyes, dull skin and dark circles. Do this often enough and you can see how endless sleepless nights can add up to a less than beautiful reflection in the mirror.

HOW IT HAPPENS – A DECADE-BY-DECADE GLANCE AT SKIN AGEING

THIRTIES

This third decade of our life is when we start to see the first signs that we truly are entering our adult years. That's when certain aspects start showing up more, like puffiness under the eyes. Granted, some people have a genetic tendency to exhibit some of this puffiness, but overall it's a sign of ageing. Meanwhile on the upper part of the eyes, there might be some excess skin and the eyebrow starts to droop a little bit. There might be a little fat accumulation in the neck and the skin might lose a bit of its youthful radiance.

Luckily, you can slow it all down by protecting yourself from further bombardment of sun damage. This is also a good time to incorporate a retinol product into your regime, which will boost your collagen reserves.

FORTIES

The picture starts to get a bit more dire. Expect to see further loss of elasticity in the skin and the loss of collagen and fat in the face will cause the cheeks to start heading south. The nasolabial folds, a.k.a. the smile lines, will also become more prominent. Any areas that experience a lot of movement, such as the eyes, will start to exhibit more wrinkling there. The infrastructure of the face might appear to be 'melting' a bit, and the corners of the mouth will turn down, as if you were frowning. This is also when those annoying age spots start deepening in colour.

FIFTIES AND BEYOND

During this time, the aforementioned changes become even more magnified. Again, loss of collagen and fat makes the face sag and even the bony structure of the face starts to go. If you think of your skin as a sofa, the collagen within it can be compared to the cushy filling and as it decreases, the 'sofa' deflates and sags. At this point, a facelift would do a nice job of redraping all of this loose skin, but it can't replace the fullness that has been lost.

CHAPTER THREE
ON THE HOMEFRONT

Few can disagree that, regardless of your starting point, a well-rounded, high-quality and consistent skin care regime is the most crucial factor in achieving and maintaining the skin of your dreams. Your genes might have predetermined your skin type, but that doesn't mean that you have to live with skin that is less than flawless.

Admittedly, devising and ultimately sticking to the ideal skin care regime is a pretty tall order. We live in a time when newness is valued above all else, relegating today's hot property into tomorrow's old news, often long before you've had a chance to get to know what it was all about. The skin care scene has also drastically changed; classics like cleansers and toners have been joined by a multitude of products that claim to exfoliate, purify, detoxify, lighten and even amplify. Sometimes a single product professes to do all of these things on its own! Factor in the countless skin care brands crowding department store shelves, all claiming to be the latest and greatest beauty innovation, and it becomes easy to see how such confusion can arise.

It doesn't have to be this way. Buying mounds of products that don't deliver on their promises doesn't have to be an accepted occurrence. Neither should perpetual confusion over what types of products will produce the best results for your specific skin type. The last twenty years have brought about significant advances in the skin care industry and – surprise, surprise – a lot of them actually come through on their claims. Narrowing it all down is a matter of being informed on what actually works and what is just selling a pipe dream.

If I were to peek in my patients' medicine cabinets, I'm sure I'd be greeted with enough skin care products to moisturise a small foreign nation. Yet, I know that a lot of women are still searching for that magical product that truly works. (I know this because I hear it

31

constantly in my practice.) While I don't think there is such a thing
as a magic elixir – ageing is inevitable, after all – I do believe that
preventing flaws is far easier than fixing them. By this I mean that it's
crucial to select skin care products based on basic criteria, such as
ingredients that are proven to improve the skin, properly assessing
the condition of your skin, your goals, and what is within the realm
of realistic expectations. If you are in your 30s, maybe it's time
to stop wishing for the skin of a teenager.

As a dermatologist, I have a lot of tools at my disposal to help the
skin look its best but, contrary to popular opinion, I'm not a magician.
Rather, I like to think of myself as my patients' partner, educating and
guiding them towards an effective skin care routine that will maintain
their skin as healthy and radiant as possible. We've come a long way
with developing doctor's office techniques that can easily and
dramatically rejuvenate the skin, but that's only half of the beautifying
equation. What a patient puts on her skin day in and day out is key – so
much so that I can easily differentiate between my patients who are
faithful to their cleansers, moisturisers, eye creams and the rest who
disregard my advice, usually on the assumption that I can easily fix
everything. But honestly, what's the point of those pricey visits to the
dermatologist and to your beloved beauty therapist if you aren't
maintaining all of their hard work at home? I like to compare it to
maintenance of the teeth: you continue to brush and floss long after
a visit to the dentist, right? The same commitment should be devoted
to your complexion.

In this chapter I will guide you through the dizzying product
maze and along the way blast the perception that a skin care routine
has to be complicated and time-consuming in order to truly make

a difference to your skin's appearance. Also, at the end of the chapter,
I will provide a detailed list of all of the ingredients that I consider
to be among the most innovative and impactful.

TREAT WHAT AILS YOU

PROBLEM: HYPERPIGMENTATION

It's sometimes cute (freckles) and sometimes not (spotting on
chest and hands) but this much is true: hyperpigmentation is one
of the most common complaints today.

Most types of pigment changes in the skin can be attributed to two
major factors: hormonal shifts (pregnancy and the use of oral
contraceptives are likely culprits) and prolonged exposure to the sun.
A skin injury, disease or cosmetic procedure might also contribute
to this uneven accumulation of skin pigment in the form of post-
inflammatory hyperpigmentation. When the cause is hormonal, the
pigmentation is called melasma and it shows up as irregularly shaped
blotches, usually on the cheeks, forehead and upper lip. It's a very
common condition but, unfortunately, one of the most difficult to get
rid of. A few lucky patients might see it go away on its own.

Solar lentigos are also known as sun spots and, despite what many
believe, ageing is not the cause – our dear friend the sun is.
Take a peek at an elderly person's naked body and you'll see that
the vast spotting on her face and hands doesn't exist on her
sun-protected areas.

Solution

All types of hyperpigmentation issues benefit greatly from at-home bleaching products. Look for proven bleaching agents, like kojic acid, in your skin care products. When combined with retinoids and glycolic acid, which work largely by exfoliating the skin, these bleaching products tend to be even more efficient.

Above all else, it's crucial that you become fanatical about sun avoidance. There is no other condition that is as aggravated by sunlight. Need to step outside? Then by all means do so, but not without loading up on a sunscreen that blocks both UVA and UVB rays.

What you can expect . . .

Given time to work, this regime can significantly fade most types of hyperpigmentation, although those due to hormonal issues are usually more challenging to treat.

Supplement it with . . .

If there is one condition that lasers are superb at treating, it's hyperpigmentation. Lasers such as the *Q-switch ruby*, *Alexandrite* and *Nd:Yag* are great choices and can bring about quick results. Certain chemical peels, including the *TCA peel*, are very helpful, too. (We discuss all of these in-office procedures in *Chapter Six: Radiance Revealed*.)

PROBLEM: ACNE

Everyone breathes a huge sigh of relief when they've passed their teenage years, confident that their days of fighting acne are gone forever. I hate to say it, but I actually treat more adult acne than I do adolescent acne. Its presence is very distressing to patients, and they are often clueless as to how to rid themselves of it.

In adults, acne can often be traced to a hormonal imbalance, but there are other culprits, such as stress. Quite simply, acne is the result of the pore (or hair follicle) becoming blocked by exfoliated skin cells that are never thoroughly expelled. Instead, the shed cells stick together inside the pore and this plug, along with the accompanying sebum, then becomes a source of nutrition for bacteria. The bacteria can then invade the pore and cause inflammation. In all, not a pretty picture.

Solution

Now for the good news: with the many acne treatments that are available today, adult acne can soon be as distant a memory as your school photo. Topping the list of wonder ingredients are retinoids, which are derivatives of vitamin A that work by controlling the cell stickiness that is the primary cause of acne. The most popular retinoid is tretinoin, and it can be found in the prescription medications *Retin-A* and *Retin-A Micro*. Other retinoids are tazarotene (found in the prescription medication *Tazorac*) and to a slightly lesser degree retinol, which is found in many products sold 'over the counter'.

One can get significant improvement by unclogging the pore, and salicylic acid, a beta hydroxy acid that is lipid soluble and can therefore penetrate the sebaceous material in the follicle, is simply magical.

Salicylic acid is found in a number of products, even cleansers. Finally, it's very helpful to use a topical antibiotic, such as *Benzamycin*, to control the presence of bacteria and the role that they play.

Supplement it with . . .
An in-office salicylic or glycolic acid peel, administered every couple of weeks, is an excellent partner to an acne-blasting home routine.

What you can expect . . .
As long as the patient is commited to a maintenance programme, acne is a very treatable condition. Patience, at least eight weeks' worth, is crucial, since the skin needs time to regenerate into a healthier version of itself.

PROBLEM: FROM FINE LINES TO FURROWS

Ah, wrinkles. They may as well be the mascot for ageing, since they are the focus of pretty much every skin care advertisement. For a woman, this preoccupation is likely to start in her late 20s to early 30s, when she spots that first indication that she's no longer a teenager. From there, it only gets more substantial, but there are ways to slow it down.

Solution
Keep the skin amply hydrated, as any kind of dryness may exaggerate wrinkles. Products with retinoic acid are proven to increase collagen production, which will in turn alleviate wrinkling. Ask your dermatologist for a prescription.

What you can expect . . .

Once a wrinkle has made itself comfortable on your skin, it's pretty difficult to remove it altogether. (Hence, my 'prevention is everything' motto of skin care!) But, if you start early enough, and become vigilant in avoiding wrinkle-causing sun damage and stick to a consistent routine, you can expect those critters to become softer and more diffused.

PROBLEM: SENSITIVE AND IRRITATED SKIN

Sometimes, identifying your specific skin condition can turn into a guessing game that you seem to never have the answer to. One of the best examples of this form of mistaken identity is skin that is irritated and overly sensitive. Since redness and peeling, usually around the nose and forehead, are characteristic of sensitive and irritated skin, it is often brushed off as being dry. In reality, this type of skin is brought on by a genetic condition that can become worse, usually while you're under stress.

Solution

The very first step in controlling sensitive and irritated skin is to calm the skin down. This can be accomplished with soaps that contain zinc as well as with a low-dose hydrocortisone cream. Botanical ingredients like rosemary and aloe are also fantastic at naturally relaxing the skin. A standard regime involves using such ingredients for a month. After the skin has normalised it can then tolerate more active ingredients that in the past weren't a viable option for such sensitive skin.

What you can expect . . .

The peeling, rough texture will be vastly improved and the uncomfortable tightness alleviated.

PROBLEM: UNEVEN TEXTURE AND LOSS OF RADIANCE

More often than not, what stands between 'good' skin and 'amazing' skin is the surface texture. Amazing skin has a lot going for it, but the main factor is how smooth and velvety it is. Babies' skin is often synonymous with this, and while we might never get back to that point, it is entirely possible to take a few steps back.

Solution

The first step is to analyse why the skin is now uneven and rough to the touch. In most cases, the culprit is an accumulation of dead skin cells that haven't been properly removed. The key word here is 'exfoliation'. Look for products containing alpha and beta hydroxy acids, namely glycolic and salicylic acid. Depending on how much your skin can tolerate, you can devise a complete programme around these active ingredients. I know that many cleansers feature these acids, but in my opinion, they work best in a product that will remain on your skin. If the dullness is a result of hyperpigmentation, then a bleaching product would be a great addition.

What you can expect . . .

Like with everything else, patience is the word of the day. Your imperfections didn't happen overnight, so you can't expect them to disappear overnight. After at least a month on a regular regime, you can expect to have substantially smoother and glowing skin.

HOW TO IMPROVE YOUR SKIN IN . . .

ONE WEEK

The clock is ticking, but don't despair; there's plenty that you can do in just seven days to make your skin the very best in can be. The magic word here is 'exfoliation' and granular scrubs, pore cleansing clay masks and glycolic and salicylic acid do the job like no other. An effective regime can consist of a mask every few nights, followed by either a salicylic acid product to clean the pores and glycolic acid to remove dead skin cells. Remember to top it off with an appropriate hydrating product afterwards.

ONE MONTH

The previous salicylic/glycolic/mask/scrub combination offers you a great headstart and you can now supplement it with a retinol product. Experiment with different versions until you find one that your skin can tolerate. I guarantee that it will be worth the effort, since nothing improves the condition of your pores and gives skin such a beautiful clarity like this vitamin A derivative. Finally, prevent a barely visible spot from becoming a darker one by adding a bleaching ingredient.

THE BOTTOM LINE

All of the answers to your most burning questions.

WHAT IS A 'CLINICAL RESULT' AND WHY SHOULD I CARE?

As a physician, I'm trained to cast a critical eye on all types of statistics
and supposed success rates that don't have solid research behind
them. Whenever a beauty company quotes a level of improvement with
their latest product after a certain number of weeks, it doesn't quite
paint the full picture. In other words, the public is never told just how
many participants were in the study, or even what the condition of the
skin was to begin with.

   That said, it doesn't necessarily mean that every quoted percentage
of improvement is full of dead air. The bottom line is: don't believe
everything you hear just because it's in a lively commercial with a
gorgeous twenty-year-old model.

IS A £200 CREAM WORTH EVERY PENNY?

What is it about creams with astronomical price tags that make
perfectly sane women, and a handful of men, too, run to the stores to
stock up on them? Judging from my patients' testimonials, a lot of this
brouhaha is wildly undeserved. But let's face it – there's something
very exciting about buying a luxurious cream with the price tag to
match, but any informed consumer will see past the glamour appeal.

   To be fair, it is sometimes necessary to place a higher price tag on
certain creams simply because better ingredients are more expensive.

Some of the chain store own-label brands, for example, can't make use of certain raw ingredients because it would simply cost too much, an expense that they would have to share with their customers.

DOES ANYTHING TRULY HELP WITH COLLAGEN PRODUCTION?

The master of all selling points in beauty advertising has got to be one that promises increased collagen production. And with the critical role that collagen plays in the beauty of the skin, it's not that difficult to understand why. I hate to be the one to deliver this news, but the only ingredient known to stimulate collagen production is retinoid, famously found in *Retin-A* and *Renova*. The scientific data behind retinoid has proven that it penetrates deep into the dermal layer where the collagen resides. Other studies have also demonstrated, with less definitive results, that vitamin C can increase collagen synthesis.

ARE THESE PORES MINE FOREVER?

They're as annoying as mosquitoes on a summer night but, unfortunately, the 20,000 pores that are spread out across your face can't simply be swatted away. Basically, people with oily skin tend to have larger pores than those with normal to dry skin, but large pores and oily skin don't necessarily go hand in hand.

   An excess of large pores often results in skin that looks rough and uneven. As we age and lose collagen, this decreased elasticity results in the enlargement of the pores. I always explain it to my patients in this way. Think of a straw (the pore) floating upright in a puddle of jelly (the skin). As the jelly starts to melt, the straw loses its balance. Using this analogy, it makes sense that stimulating the collagen in the skin can result in firmer skin and a smaller pore.

Pores can never be eradicated permanently, but a combination of alpha hydroxy and glycolic acid can help them be less prominent.

ROUTINE MATTERS

The bare essentials of at-home skin care.

CLEANLINESS COUNTS

Today's cleansers are a sophisticated bunch, as they not only remove the day's grime but can also provide tangible and long-lasting benefits. Someone with acne-prone skin, for example, might do well with an exfoliating cleanser containing glycolic or salicylic acid. Even though a cleanser remains in contact with the skin for barely a minute, in that short time it will have prepped the skin to receive an exfoliating cream. Better penetration of the cream will be achieved simply because of the cleanser. Similarly, botanicals such as green tea are extremely soothing, and a cleanser that is chock-full of such ingredients is beneficial for those with sensitive skin types.

As a general rule, those with dry skin should opt for a creamy cleanser that has very little foaming action; oily skin does well with gel cleansers, and those lucky enough to have normal skin can use pretty much anything. Cleansing twice a day is ideal but if you must

absolutely whittle it down to just once daily, I recommend that it be
done at night. It's been said a million times, but going to sleep with
a face full of make-up is an open invitation to spots and dull skin.

TONE

There's just something about toners that people really love. Toners
are actually relics of the days when most cleansers left heavy residue
on the skin and one needed to remove it with this extra step. Today's
cleansers pretty much clean up after themselves, so a toner with
strong astringent actions is unnecessary, not to mention dehydrating.
A benefit is derived, however, from using a toner that is formulated
with active ingredients, such as antioxidants. If you choose to use such
a toner for these benefits, just keep in mind that the percentage of
active ingredients in a toner isn't as high as you'd find in a cream.

MOISTURISE

There's something comforting about a moisturiser, even if it's just
because they're such a traditional part of the skin grooming process.
Pretty much every complexion can benefit from a moisturiser, even
an oily skin.

   Moisturisers don't erase years off your age, but they perform
another function that is almost as important: they keep your skin
hydrated. As the uppermost level of the skin, the *stratum corneum*,
confronts a daily assault from the environment, a moisturiser works
by creating a barrier between your skin and the air. Without this
barrier, the skin would flake and get irritated.

Of course, many of today's popular moisturisers, whether oil-based or water-based, don't just hydrate. (And besides, where's the sex appeal in that?) A moisturiser containing antioxidants, such as vitamin C and green tea, performs a double duty by adding an extra source of protection against free radical damage from UV radiation from the sun and other environmental influences.

PROTECT

Without a doubt, positively and absolutely, there is no product more important in the health and beauty of your skin than sunblock. If I had my way, I'd get rid of the sun altogether – that's how detrimental it is. But in the real world, a sunblock is the second best choice and it should be considered as essential as your toothpaste and toothbrush. Several studies have been done on identical twins who have followed different lifestyles and in case after case, it's been proven that the twin who diligently protected her skin had far less damage than her careless sibling.

An easy way to incorporate sun protection into your lifestyle is to use cosmetics with a built-in sun protection factor (SPF). Just take note that a study recently showed that these types of products tend to shift around the face and seep into the follicles in the skin, quickly losing their potency in about two hours. My preferred choice is to slather a separate sunblock with a minimum SPF 15 every day, prior to heading outside.

(For more on the role that the sun has in ageing, please refer to *Chapter Two: What Ages Us?*)

EXTRA, EXTRA

EXFOLIATION

Sometimes, even a sophisticated organ like the skin needs a bit
of assistance in performing what should come naturally. Exfoliation,
the act of loosening the dead skin cells from the upper layer of the
skin, has risen in prominence and with good reason. That accumulated
debris dulls the complexion, particularly as we age and our cell
turnover process slows down. Regular use of an exfoliant, either in a
scrub or via an exfoliating agent like glycolic and salicylic acid, helps
the skin along. It also allows better penetration of the moisturiser
that follows it, and is a must prior to self-tanning.

It is easy to become over zealous with exfoliating. If a granular
scrub is your preferred tool, then choose one with perfectly spherical
particles that don't scratch the skin. Also, don't rub too vigorously.
When it comes to exfoliating, it is possible to have too much of
a good thing.

EYE CREAMS

Surely you've been lectured on how the eye area is the most delicate on the face and should be carefully tended to? But, if you're like many harassed patients that I treat, an eye cream is usually the first part of the routine to go flying out the window. This is a big, big mistake.

The eye area suffers from a lot of cosmetic problems. It gets wrinkled easily, might have some crêpiness and a proliferation of visible blood vessels that show up as darkness under the eyes. It might also be more sensitive than the rest of the face and become easily irritated. And since it has scant oil glands, it often dries up considerably.

For all of these reasons, an eye cream is an absolute essential. Even better would be one with a built-in sunscreen for an extra dose of protection. Look for formulas with the most potent moisturising and wrinkle-fighting ingredients. If you're truly lacking the time or the inclination, then go ahead and use your moisturiser in this area. Hey, that's what I do!

BEAUTY FIRST AID KIT

SOMETIMES, DESPITE DOING ALL OF THE RIGHT THINGS TO KEEP YOUR COMPLEXION FLAWLESS, A BEAUTY DISASTER WILL SHOW UP UNANNOUNCED. ENSURE THAT INTRUDERS LIKE PUFFY EYES, DULL SKIN AND BLEMISHES DISAPPEAR AS QUICKLY AS THEY ARRIVE BY KEEPING YOUR 'BEAUTY FIRST AID KIT' FULLY STOCKED. THE FOLLOWING FIVE INGREDIENTS ARE ALL THAT YOU NEED:

1. Green tea bags
2. Brown sugar
3. Milk
4. Ice
5. Clay face mask

DE-PUFF YOUR EYES

Moisten green tea bags with water and chill them in the refrigerator for a few minutes. Lie down with the chilled bags over your eyes. The polyphenols in the green tea acts as an anti-inflammatory and the cooling reduces swelling.

INSTANT RADIANCE

Grind brown sugar with warm milk and let the mixture cool to room temperature. This is a great scrub since it exfoliates in two ways: the lactic acid in the milk acts as a mild exfoliant and the sugar granules deliver a scrubbing action.

DEFLATE A SPOT

When a blemish is really red and inflammed, an ice cube placed over it will instantly calm it down. Follow that with a dab of a clay face mask to dry out the pimple.

ROUTINE ODDS AND ENDS

ORDERLY FASHION

First you cleanse, then you tone – you'd be surprised at how many people still get that wrong!

But seriously, the order of products is determined by how many, and what types, of products comprise your routine. For example, I often advise my patients to use a vitamin A product, like prescription retinoids or over-the-counter retinols, only at night. These powerful ingredients tend to make the skin extra sensitive to light and can leave your skin terribly burned if not properly protected. Also, the sun can decrease the ingredients' efficacy.

Protective antioxidants, such as green tea, grape seed extracts and vitamin C are ideal for daytime use. If a bleaching product is a part of your routine, you can safely add it on top. Top it all off with a moisturiser, if necessary.

If your routine incorporates several active ingredients, it's best not to use them simultaneously. Some skin care brands emphasise the combination of actives like glycolic and salicylic acids, for example, within the same product. This, however, isn't a beneficial attribute, since they need to work more efficiently at different concentrations and their combined appearance in a single product might cause them to inactivate each other.

PATIENCE, PATIENCE, PATIENCE . . .

At the start of any new skin care regime, the prospect of flawless skin can leave us giddy with excitement. As days go by and that dream skin has yet to make an appearance, it's easy to become discouraged and fling those products in the bin, only to start all over again with a new assortment of products. This is all understandable – and I've seen it dozens of times with my patients – but trust me when I say that it'll all pay off in the end.

New products, particularly those with collagen-stimulating properties, need ample time to work; there's no way that this can be accomplished overnight. I advise that people try out their new products for at least a month (two or three months is actually ideal, but I know how impatient we can all be) before moving on to the next thing. The fact is that you aren't going to see any improvement in your skin after just a few days. Those products that exfoliate the surface of the skin will give you a faster result.

GLOSSARY

COSMECEUTICALS

You're probably very familiar with cosmeceuticals, even if it's the first time you've heard such a word. Famed dermatologist Albert Kligman, MD coined the term and, without a doubt, the advent of skin care products featuring these types of ingredients – from retinol and alpha hydroxy acids to vitamin C – has revolutionised the way skin behaves and looks. Traditionally, a drug has been defined as a substance that can treat and prevent disease, or bring about a change in the body. On the opposite end of the spectrum are cosmetics, which are classified as inert substances that only cleanse or enhance the skin. Cosmeceuticals fall somewhere within this gray area and their ability to bring a significant and tangible change to the skin is the real deal.

That said, however, the extensive list of benefits that these products promise to deliver should be taken with a pinch of salt. With the exception of retinoids, none of these claims have been evaluated by the relevant governing bodies. To do so requires a process that is almost comparable to sending a few trainee astronauts to the moon; it's a process so exhausting and costly that most skin care companies decide to soften their claims and do without this endorsement.

Now that you know what a cosmeceutical is, let's talk about what a cosmeceutical does. And that, in one word, is plenty. Pretty much everyone can benefit from a cosmeceutical product. Actually, you might have already indulged and never even realised it. Here are a few cosmeceutical 'superstars' proven to deliver myriad benefits, from smoothing lines and wrinkles to imparting a healthy glow.

VITAMIN A

Tretinoin

If you're starting to not love your reflection in the mirror, then a vitamin A product is one of the best investments you could make for yourself. Years of scientific research have proven that certain vitamin A derivatives, known as retinoids, can significantly improve accumulated sun damage and even help with chronological (non-sun-induced) ageing. Tretinoin is the most well-documented retinoid and it can be found in *Retin-A*, *Retin-A Micro* and *Renova*.

Some irritation, in the form of redness and flakiness, is normal upon initial use, but it tends to clear up soon after. Expect to see a reduction in fine lines and wrinkles in approximately three months.

Types of retinoids available by prescription only

···》Tretinoin – in *Retin-A*, *Retin-A Micro* and *Renova*; approved for acne and photodamage
···》Adapalene – in *Differin*
···》Tazarotene – in *Tazorac/Zorac*; less irritating than tretinoin

Retinol

Years after retinoids (in the form of *Retin-A*) hit the market, the mad scientists at many beauty companies started tinkering with a version for 'over-the-counter' usage. The result was retinol, a close relation to tretinoin that must first be converted to retinaldehyde and then to all-trans retinoic acid in the skin. Like its distant relatives, retinol is said to simulate collagen, unclog pores, promote a rosy glow and help

with acne and rosacea. Even more so than with tretinoin, retinol
can sometimes be highly irritating to the skin.

THE ACIDS

The word 'acid' might alarm some people, but be assured that these
naturally occurring acids are unbeatable at accelerating the cell
renewal process. Meet the family:

- Alpha Hydroxy Acid (AHA) – glycolic (sugarcane); malic (apples);
  tartaric (grapes); lactic (sour milk); citric (citrus fruits). Ideal for
  removing surface dead skin cells.
- Beta Hydroxy Acid (BHA) – salicylic acid, the lone BHA, is found
  naturally in willow bark, sweet birch bark and wintergreen leaves.
  It is a fat-soluble acid, allowing it to penetrate into the pores.
- Poly Hydroxy Acid (PHA) – a newer, less iritating acid, that is
  easily tolerated by most complexions

BOTANICAL GARDEN

Their roots are embedded in the past, but botanical ingredients –
such as those from plants and flowers – are the most modern way
to get a beautiful complexion. I personally like them for their proven
healing, hydrating and antiseptic properties. Also, when combined
with active dermatological ingredients, botanicals can help take
some of the sting away.

Here are a few of my personal favourites.

Aloe	Palmarosa
Camellia	Rice brand
Chamomile	Rosemary
Cypress	Shea butter
Geranium	Squalene
Lavender	Tea tree oil
Liquorice	Witch hazel
Maté	Ylang-ylang
Oakmoss	

ANTIOXIDANTS / THE VITAMINS

It is such a vicious cycle that it's hard to believe that it's one that most people happily bring upon themselves. I'm talking about sun damage, often glamorously referred to as sunbathing. When the sun's ultraviolet rays, UVA and UVB, hit the skin, the process of skin destruction is immediately activated. If the skin's natural reserves of antioxidant ingredients are ample enough, this process can sometimes be slowed down significantly. Naturally, using a skin care line rich in numerous antioxidants is a step in the right beautifying direction.

I will be reviewing some of the most proven antioxidants, such as green tea extract, grape seed extract and vitamin C. Others include: vitamin A, coenzyme Q10, lycopene and alpha lipoic acid.

GREEN TEA EXTRACT

Green tea is proving to be as potent on the skin as it is inside the body. The data that has been released on the powers of green tea is just too impressive to ignore. I was already a believer and I had already incorporated a high amount into my skin care line, but after reading up on the latest data, I decided to boost the levels of green tea in the products.

A lot of the medical studies that have been released on green tea show that when applied on the skin it protects it from ultraviolet light and may even help prevent skin cancer. In the medical field, daily oral intake of green tea helps to prevent prostate cancer.

GRAPE SEED EXTRACT

Contains powerful antioxidants that can prevent and repair oxidative stress.

VITAMIN C

Famous for its instability, vitamin C is still a potent antioxidant. The version featured in most products is ascorbic acid, which is also found in human skin. Ultraviolet radiation lowers the skin's ascorbic acid reserve, compromising the amounts needed for collagen production.

VITAMIN E

Topical application of vitamin E may reduce adverse responses to the sun, such as redness and swelling.

THE WHITENERS

If spotting is your concern, then you're surely familiar with this group of skin lighteners. Here are the top whitening ingredients:

···> hydroquinone – a chemical that is used in low concentrations, usually 2% for over-the-counter products and 4% in prescription formulas.
···> natural alternatives – mulberry extract, liquorice, thyme extracts, kojic acid and azelaic acid.

NEW NAMES ON THE BLOCK

The jury is still out on a lot of these new ingredients, but they're certainly worth noting:

···> Copper
···> Kinetin – a plant and yeast growth hormone said to slow the ageing process
···> Human growth factors
···> Omega 3 oils – essential fatty acids are key in nutrition, unsure if the same logic applies to topical skin care
···> Olive oil – great on bread, said to be nourishing on the skin

TOP TEN QUESTIONS
TO ASK A DOCTOR

What is the doctor trained in? Is he or she trained in dermatology (which is the ideal) or something unrelated?

Is the doctor board-certified in his field? You'd be surprised at how many doctors are not board-certified, so that you miss out on the extra training and knowledge this certification represents.

What specific training has the doctor had in the types of procedures he or she administers? Additional training isn't mandatory, but it's always a bonus.

Are cosmetic dermatology treatments the primary focus of the doctor's practice? Or is a procedure like *Botox* something that he or she does only occasionally?

What kind of results can I expect? An honest doctor will tell you what results are realistic.

How many treatments will I need to achieve my desired results?

How often will I have to come in for maintenance?

What are the potential side effects from my chosen procedure?

Does the doctor have any 'before' and 'after' pictures that he or she can share with you? It's always helpful to see real people who have undergone such procedures, even in Polaroid photos.

What is this going to cost me? Ask for a detailed list of prices, including all those hidden fees. Keep in mind that a 'name' doctor who practises in a large city might be pricier than one from a smaller town.

PART TWO

BEAUTY OPTIONS AND TECHNIQUES

CHAPTER FOUR
BRING ON THE *BOTOX*

I'm often asked what I consider to be the greatest advancement in cosmetic dermatology and without hesitation I say, 'Botox'. The advent of treating wrinkles with *Botox* injections has allowed doctors like myself to treat conditions that in the past not even plastic surgery could remedy. Don't like the way that your forehead stays furrowed long after you've stopped worrying? Then shoot those lines into oblivion. What about those little lines around your eyes that are still in existence despite your fanatical use of eye cream? Shoot some *Botox* there, too. And whatever happened to your regal neck? Yes, *Botox* will bring back your beloved neck, as well. All of this improvement with no recovery period, minimal pain and extremely natural results.

Botox has many uses, but its claim to fame is how well it smoothes dynamic wrinkles. Also known as 'wrinkles in motion', these lines are most often found across the forehead, between the brows and around the eyes. Constant frowning is one sure way to get them, but any sort of movement will bring them on, including laughing heartily and squinting at your computer screen. In other words, just being alive brings them on. What happens over time is that the line morphs from a 'wrinkle in motion' to the more dreaded 'wrinkle in action'. Like it or not, that little guy is there to stay.

For a substance with such dramatic beautifying properties, *Botox* has a much publicised and controversial background. *Botox*, or 'botulinum toxin type A', is a highly purified derivative of a toxin that in much, much larger doses could be hazardous. When used for cosmetic, or wrinkle zapping, purposes the toxin is purified and diluted and injected into the facial muscles. Almost instantly, the toxin blocks the nerve impulses that control muscle movement by restricting the patient's abilities to contract the facial muscles. No contraction of the muscle equals no movement of the skin lying over it and no movement equals no wrinkles. A smoothing effect is seen while the patient is still in the exam chair, with improvement continuing over the following couple of days. This result lasts approximately three to six months, at which point most patients gradually return to their original state of wrinkling.

Of the seven different forms of the *botulinum* toxin that exist, type A is the one that is most studied and used and the only one approved for the cosmetic treatment of frown lines. *Neurobloc*, manufactured by Elan Pharmaceuticals, is another paralysing agent, this time derived from *botulinum* type B. It is used very similarly to *Botox*, but it's only approved for cervical dystonia, which are involuntary contractions of the neck and shoulders. However, the potential of *Neurobloc* as a cosmetic treatment is starting to emerge, with more information to come within the next couple of years.

The immobilising properties that make *Botox* sound potentially morbid are the same ones that make it an incredible drug. During the 1980s, researchers discovered that these properties were of tremendous benefit for patients suffering from involuntary muscle spasms associated with illnesses such as cerebral palsy. Compared to the other treatments available at the time, such as muscle relaxants, *Botox* was found to be the most effective since it worked quickly and had minimal side effects. In 1989 *Botox* was approved for the treatment of strabismus (commonly known as 'crossed eyes') and blepharospasm (involuntary winking). The following year *Botox* was granted another approval, this time for cervical dystonia.

The story of how *Botox* transformed from a medical drug to one with myriad beauty benefits is as fascinating as *Botox* itself. An ophthalmologist in Canada, Dr Jean Carruthers, noticed that the patients whom she was treating with *Botox* were not only seeing an improvement with their medical conditions, but the wrinkles in the surrounding areas were virtually disappearing. Intrigued by this development, Dr Carruthers mentioned it to her husband, who happened to be a dermatologist. Just as intrigued, the dermatologist began to try out *Botox* on his patients, starting with his thirty-year-old receptionist with deep creases between her eyebrows, and arrived at the same conclusion as his wife. A few years later, in 1990, the first medical paper was written on the potential of *Botox* as a significant aid in the field of cosmetic dermatology, bringing *Botox* greater recognition and acceptance among cosmetic dermatologists.

The buzz on *Botox* started to spread and I became among the first in my field to partake in this exciting development. At the time, a lot of my patients were frightened of *Botox* and all of its perceived dangers. And to be honest, I can understand these fears. There's something slightly alarming about telling a patient that I'm going to erase their wrinkles with a shot of something that originates from a toxin!

The fact is that nobody has been harmed by *Botox* or even had an allergic reaction to it – much less died from it. Research has shown that in humans, a lethal injection would consist of 2,500 to 3,000 units of *Botox*. For patients suffering from the muscle spasms associated with cerebral palsy, to mention just one example, dosages as high as 1,000 units are used quite routinely. And when *Botox* is used for cosmetic reasons the average dosage is – drum roll, please – up to 75 units. That's paltry and insignificant and most importantly to you, *extremely* safe.

Once their concerns were assuaged, the next question was the all-important, How will I look? Will I look strange and oddly frozen? Will others detect my little secret? Even today, one of the biggest misconceptions about *Botox* is that it will eliminate all facial expressions. This theory is so widespread that even Hollywood directors have put their oar into the *Botox* debate, arguing that *Botox* has robbed their actresses of the ability to emote. I've certainly seen my fair share of expressionless faces, but with as much *Botox* as I administer in a day, I can vouch for how natural *Botox* can look. With the proper technique, an artistic eye and a conservative approach, the patient should look like themselves, only more refreshed and rejuvenated.

Almost a decade after *Botox* landed on the scene, a spotless record of success has finally earned it approval from the UK authorities for treating moderate to severe wrinkling in the glabellar lines, commonly referred to as frown lines. These two grooves are parallel to one another above the bridge of the nose and, over time, they tend to become deeper and more prominent. Of course, the potential of *Botox* isn't limited to this one area. Governing bodies dictate that a drug must prove its safety and effectiveness through clinical trials, and even though *Botox* has myriad uses, each of these uses has to present this proof and the approval is awarded per application. For example, *Botox* is extremely effective at erasing (albeit temporarily) crow's-feet and the bands on the forehead, so those are the areas that will probably receive the next approval for cosmetic use. In the future, approvals for treating back spasms and migraines could be next. In the meantime, physicians can use *Botox* however they see fit. This is called off-label usage and it's a practice that is perfectly legal as long as the drug has been approved for something.

For now, this validation is a huge step towards bringing greater acceptance and understanding for the many conditions that can be treated with *Botox*.

With this new-found respect, however, comes a dangerous misconception that since *Botox* is a relatively quick and simple procedure, it can be done anywhere, by anyone. This couldn't be farther from the truth. Just because a *Botox* injection can be administered in less than thirty minutes doesn't make it any less serious than, say, a laser eye-correction procedure. The physicians who are best suited to administer *Botox* are trained and board-certified cosmetic dermatologists and plastic surgeons that have extensive experience with *Botox* and understand advanced facial anatomy. And surely you've heard of so-called *Botox* parties, where a group of people meet at a friend's house, alcohol is served, and *Botox* is administered in another room. If a complication were to arise, would you want a bunch of your tipsy friends cheering you on? Probably not.

Now for that crucial question, How does it look? If there's one word that sums up the result attained with *Botox*, it's 'normal'. Rested and rejuvenated are two other good adjectives, as are refreshed and replenished. Quite simply, you look exactly the same but only better. The areas that needed smoothing are smoothed, while the parts that were sagging are now uplifted. If you don't personally know someone who's been injected with *Botox* (although that is becoming increasingly hard to believe) I would suggest that you turn on your television. Or go to the movies. Or pick up a fashion magazine. I can't say with total certainty just how many celebrities have jumped on the *Botox* bandwagon, but trust me when I say that if you're over forty and in the public eye, then you've probably gone in for a little injection rejuvenation.

THE *BOTOX* FACELIFT

One of the most exciting uses for *Botox* is one that I pioneered in 1997, when I discovered that by injecting it into the cords of the neck a patient could get results that resemble those from a facelift. Allow me to explain. A facelift, despite its name, treats conditions that are exclusive to the lower half of the face, such as loose skin on the cheeks, a softened jaw line, thickened neck bands and a crinkled neck. Those who have a significant amount of sagging fat in the face and neck would get great results from a facelift but the majority of people aren't at that advanced stage of ageing just yet. For them, *Botox* in the neck would be the procedure of choice.

This usage of *Botox* is so instantly dramatic that you truly have to see it to believe it. A few quick injections of *Botox*, placed in the cords of the neck, and hey presto, the bands in the neck become less prominent, the lines there disappear and even the outer corners of the mouth get picked up slightly. Another plus – there's practically no pain associated with injecting the neck. It's a wonderfully satisfying way to use *Botox*, and patients, even those who are initially sceptical about treating their neck, are thrilled with the results. I must stress, however, that because the muscles on the lower half of the face are not as clearly defined as those on the upper part of the face, it might become difficult for an inexperienced practitioner to deliver good results in this area.

Nothing will stop ageing permanently, not even plastic surgery, so it's not uncommon for me to see patients who've already had a facelift (or two) and would like to get a slight lift without having to undergo another surgery. When they hear that *Botox* will save them that trip to the plastic surgeon's office, they're very relieved. And smartly so.

Constantly pulling back the face will not make you look any younger and will only give you that dreaded wind tunnel effect. (You know the look. It's the one that keeps people whispering after the person has left the room.)

THE *BOTOX* BROW LIFT

They say that the eyes are the windows to the soul and, while it's an old cliché, this might explain why pretty much every patient is concerned with the appearance of his or her eyes. Even patients in their 20s will ask me if plastic surgery, such as an eye lift, is the answer to their particular problem. Before I answer this, I first hand them a mirror and ask them to point out what it is about their eyes that is bothering them. If the problem is excess skin above the eyelid or bags below the eyes then surgery can definitely help but so can *Botox*.

See, when the muscles over the brows are injected with *Botox* that area immediately lifts, bringing with it any excess skin that is hanging over the eyes. Suddenly, the eyes seem bigger and more open and brighter, almost as if a light has just been turned on overhead. I refer to this phenomenon as a non-surgical brow lift. After the patient is handed back the mirror to observe the results on one side of the face, they happily exclaim that they had no idea that they could have such a result without surgery. It's not too far-fetched to predict that *Botox* could someday replace surgical brow lifts or even eye lifts – it's hard to dispute such dramatic benefits reaped with such little pain and zero recovery time.

Those new to *Botox* are fascinated by how a needle can reshape the brows, in the process opening up the eyes and subtracting years from their age. Keep in mind, though, that as thrilling as the brow lift effect can be, it's a tricky area to treat correctly. There's a fine line between rejuvenating the face and freezing it into submission and only an experienced doctor can avoid such an undesirable result. Only trust a physician who is reputed to know the difference.

My approach is customised to each patient. I start by assessing not just the patient's forehead lines but also his or her overall facial structure. Those elements give me just enough information to map out a plan. Let's say that the patient's forehead lines are very pronounced but her brow is naturally low. In that instance I wouldn't attempt to completely erase every single line, since in the process I risk lowering the brow even further, leaving the patient with an eye area that looks closed. (Or simply, with less space to apply eye shadow.) It's a delicate balance, since totally paralysing (and in the process, softening) the forehead muscles takes away the ability to elevate the brows. I feel it's more important to have open eyes and a few lines on the forehead than a totally smooth brow and lowered brow.

THE EYES HAVE IT

There's nothing like *Botox* for treating crow's-feet, those little lines that hover on the outer corner of each eye. These lines are known as dynamic wrinkles, or wrinkles in motion, and their existence is related to the constant movement of that part of the face. And like I said earlier, *Botox* is, without question, the treatment of choice for any type of movement-induced wrinkling. Plastic surgery does nothing for crow's-feet but pull them tighter and collagen injections will make them appear softer when the patient isn't animated, but daily facial expressions will bring them back in no time. As for treating them with lasers, you will see an improvement but it comes at the price of two weeks of recovery time and a risk of permanent changes in your pigmentation.

A fatty deposit under the eyes is best treated with surgery but I've found that a lot of patients, particularly those who are past forty years old, mistake a bulge right under their eye for fat. This bulge is actually an overworked muscle and believe it or not, a touch of *Botox* injected there will soften it. As bizarre as it sounds to inject your eye with *Botox*, it is very safe to do so. The only consequence is that this can round out the eye shape. (Some of my Asian patients actually consider this to be a perk.) The bottom line is: if you love your almond-shaped eyes then I wouldn't recommend this for you.

BOTOX ALL AROUND

One of the reasons why I'm such a believer in *Botox* is because its immense versatility is unmatched. New uses for it seem to surface at a daily rate and it's so satisfying when patients see results from *Botox* that they never dreamed of obtaining in such a short visit. Following are a few examples of *Botox*'s scope.

MIGRAINES

It's been proven that *Botox* helps with the debilitating condition of migraines. The reason isn't exactly clear, but I suspect that the muscle-relaxing effects of *Botox* have something to do with it. Another theory is that *Botox* has a positive effect on the pain transmitters of the face. A few years ago I treated a patient whom I thought was exaggerating when she said her headache immediately disappeared after having *Botox*. Today, however, I'm a believer in this application. Recently another patient told me that her crippling headaches had kept her home from work for two weeks and that to her, *Botox* was truly heaven sent. Even one of my nurses in my Miami office uses *Botox* for this purpose; her headaches are so severe that she often has to turn off the lights in her office and rest her head. For many, the instant relief that *Botox* delivers in just a shot or two – with relief lasting as long as four months – is far more desirable than taking an endless stream of pain medication. Of course, no one complains about the side benefits!

EXCESSIVE SWEATING

It doesn't classify as a cosmetic problem in the traditional sense, but profuse sweating (hyperhidrosis) is a big issue for a lot of people. Picture a supermodel walking down a runway with an armpit stain or a businessman sealing a deal with a clammy handshake and it becomes clear why many people are desperate for a solution. It so happens that the neurotransmitter (acetylcholine) that *Botox* affects in the face is the same one that triggers the sweat glands under the arms, in the palms of the hands, the soles of the feet and the forehead. Treating these areas with *Botox* temporarily reduces or even halts sweat production, with results lasting anywhere from six to eight months.

CHEST

Isn't it odd to see a perfectly unlined face against a chest full of lines? I think so and so do the patients whom I've treated in that area. I remember one patient in particular gushing about the thrill of waking up in the morning and not having a network of lines running in all directions across their chest.

ODDS AND ENDS

We already know that ageing causes everything to droop, but the nose, too? Unfortunately, this is also true, and as a result the nose tends to appear longer. A tiny amount of *Botox* injected in the tip of the nose can help relax the muscle that is causing the droop. Another consequence of ageing is loss of fat and muscle and in the chin this manifests itself as a dimpled 'cobblestone' effect. Again, a shot or two of *Botox* restores it quite well.

SIDE EFFECTS

By now you're probably thinking that *Botox* has to have a down side. Like with any other procedure, whether cosmetic or not, side effects are always a concern. In the case of *Botox*, the most common side effects are headaches, drooping of the eyebrow (brow ptosis), drooping of the eyelid (eyelid ptosis), double vision or the paralysis of the wrong muscles. Expect most of these side effects to clear up on their own within a few weeks. The only exception is brow ptosis, which can last for the lifespan of the *Botox*. Bruising at the site of the injection is another possible side effect. On a lighter note, picking an experienced doctor lessens your chances of winding up with any of these side effects in the first place.

TIPS OF THE *BOTOX* TRADE

Certain vitamins and medications, such as vitamin E and aspirin, can make you more prone to bruising at the injection site. Avoid them for approximately ten days before being treated with *Botox*.

It's important to remain upright for a minimum of two hours following treatment to ensure that *Botox* doesn't migrate. One of my new patients came prepared with an anti-snooze gadget created for drivers that gets tucked behind the ear. It works by emitting a loud buzzing sound whenever it senses that the head is lowering. The best part of this story is that her mother, also a patient, had given it to her!

Excessive smiling and frowning are what brought you to seek *Botox* in the first place. Funnily enough, you'll have to do a lot of both immediately after the treatment to ensure that the *Botox* binds properly.

THE *BOTOX* CONSULTATION

I've found that while patients are all too aware of their problem areas, they're usually at a loss as to which procedure will help to restore their looks. This confusion is quite understandable and it's one of the reasons why the consultation is an invaluable factor in ultimately having a fulfilling experience. When I meet a patient for the first time I'm not only listening to what they're saying, but I'm also observing their facial expressions. That, in itself, will tell me a lot. If, for example, they're constantly pursing their lips when speaking, then I know that the lines on the upper and lower lip are due to muscular contractions, making this patient an ideal candidate for *Botox*. I would then explain to them how tiny drops of *Botox* would simply relax this area, not paralyse it. Afterwards, I might suggest that they follow up with a peel or a laser treatment. The combination of treatments will assure that the area remains smooth for even longer.

WHAT A PAIN

Patients often ask me if *Botox* is a painful procedure. Like with any type of pain, different people feel it differently. Also, I've found that people are sometimes more afraid of the unknown and once they have the treatment they're surprised at how tolerable it was. Some other people, meanwhile, have a chronic fear of needles. To those folks I show them how tiny the needles are, kind of like acupuncture needles, and this comforts them. But trust me when I say that *Botox* is the best 'wash and wear' procedure out there. It can even be done on the night of a party! I recommend that a patient use a topical anaesthetic cream, usually *EMLA*, for thirty minutes before the procedure. This is an extra step but worthwhile, since it definitely decreases the sensation of pain during the procedure.

The procedure itself, consisting of a few pricks throughout the face, lasts no longer than fifteen minutes. I remember a new patient who was so afraid of the pain and would talk of nothing else. I asked her to sit back and relax and minutes later she was giddy over how comfortable it was. She even exclaimed that having her eyebrows tweezed was far more painful. After the very last shot is injected, we place ice packs over the face to decrease any discomfort and to help prevent any bruising that might come later.

THE FEAR FACTOR

Patients often ask me if *Botox* will cause their muscles to atrophy. Studies have shown that approximately six to eight months after stopping *Botox*, 80% of the muscle mass goes back to normal. The bottom line is: you're not going to lose control over your muscles. Some patients are even concerned about how *Botox* will affect their respiration, but I can guarantee that the amount of *Botox* that is used cosmetically will in no way affect this.

IS THERE SUCH A THING AS TOO MUCH *BOTOX*?

The only way that too much *Botox* becomes a problem is when an excessive amount is injected in one sitting, resulting in a frozen forehead, lowered brow and possible drooping of the eyelid. Over time, a very small group of patients will develop immunity to *Botox*, meaning that subsequent treatments won't have an effect.

WHAT CAN *BOTOX* TREAT?

Furrowed eyebrows
Forehead lines
Crow's-feet
Reduces under-eye bulge to open the eyes
Lines in the neck
Vertical 'smoker's' lines that run above and below the lips
Vertical 'marionette' lines that run from the outside corner
of the mouth to the chin
Lines on the chest
Dimpling on the chin
Excessive sweating

WHAT CAN'T *BOTOX* DO?

Enlarge the lips
Smooth nasolabial folds
Add volume to the cheeks
Fill in deep wrinkles

Whether you'd never heard of *Botox* or have been contemplating it
for a while now, just remember that *Botox* delivers maximum results
with the smallest amount of recuperation possible. You'll still look
like yourself, only a more refreshed, more energised version.

CHAPTER FIVE
FILLER UP

The world of cosmetic dermatology is littered with moments – those who saw the movie *The First Wives' Club* will probably remember Goldie Hawn's over-inflated lips. With such exaggerated examples it's easy to see why the concept of correcting facial flaws by injecting them with a foreign substance can seem like modern day madness. In reality, however, the category of 'fillers' is an extremely valid one, as it's the most effective way to improve a long list of skin woes. From softening the appearance of wrinkles and scars to restoring youthful volume to the face – and even giving lips that sexy 'oomph' that you've only dreamed about – fillers should be in everyone's anti-ageing arsenal.

The concept of filler materials dates back to the nineteenth century, when researchers discovered that fat taken from a patient's body was ideal for fixing facial defects. By the early 1900s, paraffin – yes, as in wax – was experimented with, only to fall out of favour twenty years later. The 1940s saw a fascination with silicone fillers, but that fad came to an end when it was discovered that silicone had an unfortunate tendency to migrate from its intended location when injected incorrectly. Improved versions of silicone are in use today and I'll discuss them later in this chapter.

In the early 1970s, a team of researchers at Stanford University in California began tinkering with bovine (cow-based) collagen. The results were very promising and finally, in 1977, the first bovine collagen injection with the trade name *Zyderm* hit the market. Its approval for use in the UK followed and today it maintains a level of unrivalled popularity. Two other versions of bovine collagen, *Zyderm II* and *Zyplast*, soon followed and, depending on the patient's needs, any of the three can be used, either exclusively or in combination.

By now you're probably asking yourself, Why from cows? First, the collagen found in cows is very similar to human collagen and as a result, only an estimated 3% of the population is allergic to it. Before any treatment, a series of skin tests spaced over a four-week period usually rule out the possibility of an allergic reaction, but even so, it's been found that 1 in 1,000 patients will experience the redness and swelling at the site of the injection associated with an allergic reaction. Fortunately, the reaction always clears up on its own and doesn't affect your general health. Secondly, and perhaps most importantly, bovine collagen delivers an extremely natural result that so far has proven difficult to replicate with a synthetic substance or even a human one.

As remarkable as bovine collagen is, however, it does have its disadvantages. The possibility of an allergic reaction, however small, still means that some people cannot use it. Also, once injected, the body quickly breaks it down and in three to six months most of the effect will have disappeared. It's easy to see how collagen injections can add up to one expensive quick fix!

Not surprisingly, attempts have been made to discover the 'perfect' filler and this endeavour has proved to be as challenging as finding the fountain of youth itself. Such a filler would have to satisfy a long list of requirements to be classified as perfect. It should be long lasting, look natural, be derived from a material that doesn't pose a risk of an allergic reaction and be easy to administer. Currently, there are a lot of promising options that meet many of these requirements, but not every single one. We will be examining these options in this chapter, as well as presenting what you can expect to see in the very near future.

ARE FILLERS FOR YOU?

A good way to determine whether you would benefit from a filler material is to study your reflection in the mirror and ask yourself the following:

> Do you have deep nasolabial folds on either side of the mouth? (These folds are also called smile lines, except that they're nothing to smile about, are they?)

> What about your forehead? Do you see a series of horizontal lines?

> Now concentrate on your mouth for a moment – do you have a multitude of tiny vertical lines above and below your lips or are the corners of your mouth turned down slightly, as if you were sulking? While you're looking at your lips consider whether you would like to replace some of the volume that time has taken away.

> Finally, does your face seem hollow and devoid of the roundness of your youth?

If, when you step away from the mirror, you have answered yes to at least one of these questions, then you're most likely an ideal candidate to be treated with a filler material.

LIP SERVICE

So many people are concerned about the appearance of their mouth
and understandably so. This area is where ageing rears its ugly head
in a significant way: the lips shrink with age and the borders of the
mouth, which function very much like a frame, tend to lose definition.
The corners of the mouth, meanwhile, turn downwards, giving the face
a sad appearance and further contributing to the marionette lines
(oral commissures) that run down to the chin.

My preferred method for restoring the integrity of the mouth is to
inject a filler material like collagen right along the borders of the lips.
A lot of women are afraid that this technique will give them lips that
are too plumped – no doubt fearing that *First Wives' Club* syndrome –
but I assure them that if done properly using only small amounts of a
filler material, this will not be the case. A great side benefit of this
technique is that the corners of the lips are lifted, bringing back that
youthful smile. I'd even say that you could easily bring the lips back to
their appearance from twenty years ago!

Another common complaint revolves around the annoying 'lipstick
bleed' lines (formally known as perioral lines) that hover directly
above and below the lips. I always tell my patients that although I could
fill in these tiny lines with a filler – and this approach would solve the
problem for a lot of patients – the perfectionist in me feels that this is
akin to painting only a portion of a room. To truly improve this area I
would suggest we fill in the borders of the lips as well. This technique
will act as a foundation for the filler that is already injected in the
upper and lower lip lines, helping it to not be broken down as quickly.

Almost daily, patients enter my office clutching a photo of the lips of

77

their dreams. I probably have enough of these photos in my office to fill another whole book! More often than not, these fantasy lips are full and luscious – Angelina Jolie is the standard-bearer for this phenomenon. Again, I try to convey to the patient that while the lips can be enhanced, the end result still has to be appropriate for their face. Nothing is worse than seeing the lips entering a room ten seconds before the person does.

First, I suggest that we subtly inject the outline of the lips. Quite often this measure gives enough of a change and the patient can choose to stop there. But, if they decide that they do indeed want something fuller, I achieve it by filling in the entire lip with the chosen filler. My goal is to have the patient leave my office with lips that look like they were born with them. An interesting footnote is the question of which lip should be fuller: top or bottom? The upper lip is often in greater need of plumping since it tends to lose the most volume, but I like the bottom lip to be slightly larger so that it forms a nice platform on which the top lip can rest.

EYE ON THE PRIZE

Dark circles under the eyes contribute greatly to that drained and fatigued look and pretty much everyone wants to know what can be done about them. The purplish hue is due to the dilated blood vessels that lie just below the surface and show through due to the area's thin and translucent skin. Elevating the under-eye area with a filler can create a new thicker layer of skin that can help to camouflage these blood vessels. This procedure will also fill in the groove around the eyes, making it markedly smoother.

SCAR FACE

Accidents and disease can leave behind unpleasant souvenirs in the form of scarring. Luckily, certain types of scars can be filled in with a filler material. A quick way to see if a specific scar would benefit from a filler is to hold the skin between the fingers and pull it taut. If the skin smoothes out with this action, then it's probably a good candidate for filling. Other types of scars, like 'ice pick' scars, cannot be successfully treated with filler materials.

WHAT CAN'T A FILLER DO?

By its very definition, a filler does not tighten the skin; so saggy jowls cannot be treated. Fillers are somewhat helpful in smoothing dynamic wrinkles, such as those commonly found on the forehead and around the eyes, but *Botox* is much better suited for this since the constant flexing of the muscle will quickly bring back that wrinkle.

I wish I could say that fillers can make those dreaded large pores a condition of the past. No such luck, as the structure of pores would result in the filler material being pushed right out.

HOW MANY FILLER MATERIALS ARE AVAILABLE TODAY?

The list of filler materials available today is long and ever changing, but bovine collagen injections are still considered the gold standard among fillers. In addition to having the longest track record of safety, bovine collagen is available in three different weights, assuring that virtually every area in need of augmentation can be treated. However, researchers are working like mad to knock bovine collagen off its very high horse and the innovations that are in this category might just accomplish this feat.

Here now, is a complete overview of fillers on the market today as well as those soon to arrive. Please note that not all of these are available in the UK at the time of printing.

BIOLOGICAL FILLERS

Materials derived from humans or animals that are naturally degraded by the body.

BOVINE COLLAGEN

Anyone who is considering collagen injections for the first time wants to know the following: Is the procedure painful? Will the collagen be bumpy under the skin? How long will the results last? And most importantly, Will I look so bad afterwards that I'll have to miss that great party?

For starters, collagen injections are one of the most comfortable procedures available thanks to the lidocaine, a local anaesthetic, that's already pre-mixed in the syringe. To make the entire process completely painless, a patient can choose to numb the area that will be treated with a thick coating of a cream that also contains lidocaine. Some patients choose to undergo the procedure without this extra step, while others happily ask for it and use the additional thirty minutes of waiting time to catch up on their magazines. The cream is then removed, the procedure performed and the skin remains numb for approximately an hour afterwards.

Some patients attest to seeing results immediately, while for others it might take three to four days for the collagen to settle into the skin. It's quite common for patients to have some redness on that first day but it is easily camouflaged with make-up. On average, patients need to return every four months to maintain the effects. This doesn't mean that the collagen has completely disappeared, but in order to maintain the original results, a touch-up is necessary. The good news is that those who start collagen treatments while still fairly young, say in their 30s, may receive near permanent results due to the constant stimulation of their own collagen.

Aside from everything you already know about bovine collagen, it's important to note that you suffer no risk of contracting BSE, or 'mad cow disease'. The company that manufactures *Zyderm* and *Zyplast*, The McGhan Medical Corp., uses cows that have been raised in an isolated ranch in California. So erase that concern from your list!

⋯⋯⟩ *Zyderm I* and *Zyderm II* – A non-cross-linked bovine collagen that is ideal for treating superficial wrinkles like horizontal forehead lines, crow's-feet and shallow scars. As I mentioned earlier, these injections are pre-mixed with lidocaine, a pain reliever, so that the procedure is minimally painful. *Zyderm II* is a more concentrated version of bovine collagen. Your doctor can help you determine which version is right for you.

⋯⋯⟩ *Zyplast* – This is cross-linked bovine collagen, meaning that the substance is thicker and more durable than *Zyderm*. It is ideal for deeper wrinkles and furrows, nasolabial folds, deep scars and to enhance the lip line.

HUMAN COLLAGEN

⋯⋯⟩ *Cosmoderm* and *Cosmoplast* (not yet available in the UK)
These two materials, also produced by McGhan Medical, are perfect examples of the innovation that exists in the area of filler materials. Comprising collagen that is derived from infant foreskin cells, *Cosmoderm* and *Cosmoplast* are considered to be the ideal form of human collagen. Ideal because it poses no risk of an allergic reaction and therefore eliminates the need for skin testing prior to treatment – a great bonus for those people who are too impatient to wait four weeks for test results before being treated. Also, its source assures it has a purity that is comparable to nothing else.

It's difficult to state with any degree of accuracy just how long the results with this filler last. Cosmetic treatments that use human collagen have not been widely used and therefore few statistics are available. However, considering that the human collagen in

Cosmoderm and *Cosmoplast* shares the same composition as bovine collagen, it might be safe to say that the duration should be similar to that of *Zyderm* and *Zyplast*. And, like with bovine collagen injections, the syringe comes pre-mixed with lidocaine for minimal discomfort. The applications of *Cosmoderm I* and *II* are similar to those of *Zyderm I* and *II*, while *Cosmoplast* equals *Zyplast* and can be used in a similar fashion.

At the time of writing this book, this material was not yet available anywhere; most likely it will be available in late 2002 or early in 2003.

HUMAN INJECTABLE TISSUE

···⋗ *Cymetra* (not yet available in the UK)

A mixture of collagen, elastin and glycosaminoglycans – three substances that are found naturally in the dermis of the skin – *Cymetra* is derived from donated human cadaver skin. An advantage of *Cymetra* is that it poses no risk of an allergic reaction and therefore the need for skin testing is eliminated. A disadvantage is that the injection is more painful than bovine collagen as there is no anaesthetic in the syringe. Also, because *Cymetra* is available in just one thickness, it lacks the versatility of other fillers. On average, its use is limited to the treatment of superficial lines and wrinkles.

⋯⋯> *Isolagen* (not yet available in the UK)
Isolagen is a material with various benefits, but speediness is definitely not among them. First, fibroblasts – the skin cells that produce collagen – are retrieved from behind the patient's ear and sent to an outside lab where they are allowed to multiply. After the cells are returned to the physician the patient has just a short window of opportunity for the cells to be injected into the skin. If too much time elapses, the cells will die and be rendered useless. It's important to remember that since fibroblasts, not collagen, are injected into the skin the patient does not leave the office with visible results. Realistically, it could take as long as four months after the treatment for enough collagen to be synthesised by the fibroblasts to see a noticeable improvement in a patient's wrinkles.

HYALURONIC ACIDS

Almost on a daily basis the question, What's new? comes up in conversations with my patients, and frequently this inquiry is directed towards the latest in filler materials. Innovation is always intriguing to patients, but they are equally interested in learning about new fillers that are long lasting and safe. My reply is that out of all the new injectable fillers that are on the horizon, I am the most excited about the hyaluronic acid family of products.

Hyaluronic acid is a polysaccharide, or natural sugar, that is crucial to the healthy functioning of the human body. The skin houses the vast majority of hyaluronic acid, with the remainder found in the muscles and skeleton. Its primary function is to provide volume and pliability to the skin and it plays a crucial role in cell growth. Interestingly enough, hyaluronic acid is commonly used in moisturisers and other cosmetics, as it is wonderfully efficient at holding onto water. An often quoted characteristic of hyaluronic acid is its capacity to bind water up to a thousand times its volume. This very property makes it ideal as a filler material, for even while a hyaluronic acid filler is being naturally degraded, what remains of the filler attracts water from the body and that function allows it to hold its shape for even longer.

In the 1960s, the first hyaluronic acid product was used for eye surgery. Today there are two families of such fillers currently available for cosmetic use. The first is created in a lab, while the other is derived from an animal source.

NON-ANIMAL HYALURONIC ACID

In 1996, the biotechnology company Q-Med of Sweden created a genetically engineered version of hyaluronic acid in the form of a clear gel called NASHA (Non-Animal Stabilised Hyaluronic Acid). This technology, which was found to be compatible with human skin, was turned into *Restylane*, an injectable filler that can be used like both collagen and fat. *Restylane* has been used extensively in Europe, Canada and South America for years now and the results so far have been extremely positive.

Several years after the introduction of *Restylane*, the company came up with two other versions: *Restylane Fine Lines* and *Perlane*. Both have the same chemical composition as the original product, but the thickness varies among the three. *Restylane Fine Lines* can be used for superficial lines anywhere on the face, such as those lines above and below the lip that lipstick always seems to bleed into. The thickest

FAT

There are more ways to inject fat than there are recipes for making stew. Although this filler has been popular for over a hundred years, positive results remain highly dependent on the experience of the doctor as well as on the technique used. First, fat is removed from the patient, usually from the lower body, and injected into the face on the same day. The remainder is kept frozen until the patient returns to the office for another treatment. Some doctors like to treat their patients once a month over a period of several months for treatments with small doses of fat. Others, meanwhile, opt to inject mega doses of fat in just one session. The downside to the latter option is the swelling and longer recuperation time; while the upside is that the results appear to be long lasting. Smaller dosages do deliver good results, but this technique doesn't seem to deliver the long-lasting results that larger doses do. The bottom line is that every doctor has his or her own method of injecting fat and accordingly, the results will vary.

Fat injections are great for enhancing volume and delivering contours to the face but they're not as effective for fine lines. Also, there is usually some swelling and bruising as the needle is larger than the one used for hyaluronic acid or collagen injections. Traditionally the fat is injected right into the patient's facial fat but some doctors are experimenting with injecting fat into the muscle and, so far, I have not seen enough positive results to be convinced of the viability of this technique. Overall, I think that the results with fat can be semi-permanent in some people and last even less than collagen in other people. Lastly, certain areas, like smile lines, seem to show greater improvement than areas like the lips.

HUMAN FASCIA (NOT AVAILABLE IN THE UK)

A medical term used to describe the thick sheets of connective tissue that line muscles, fascia has been used safely as a surgical implant for years. Recently, *Fascian* – an injectable particulate form of human fascia that is derived from human cadavers – has become available. With *Fascian*, freeze-dried particles of this connective tissue are combined with a local anaesthetic to create a dense suspension, and that is then implanted into the trouble spots. Due to its origins, some patients are concerned about the risk of disease transmission, but this risk is minimal thanks to the careful screening process that it undergoes. Finally, fascia doesn't seem to last longer than collagen.

IMPLANTS

When filler implants were introduced almost thirty years ago they brought with them great hope in being an answer to the ravages of time. In recent years, however, the initial excitement surrounding filler implants has definitely waned. High on the list of complaints is the tendency of implants to lose their original shape – they can get hard, contract and even protrude from their original location. It is also difficult to achieve the right fit because, unlike injectable fillers, implants are linear and need to conform to a certain shape. Studies are also beginning to show that implants can't be considered permanent. Ageing, as we all know, is a continuous process so what constitutes a major improvement today will be less of one in a year's time. Also, even though implants smooth certain creases really well, such as the nasolabial folds, they don't correct them entirely, making it necessary to have another filler injected over it for a complete correction.

Finally, in my experience I've found that patients want to improve their facial flaws quickly and effortlessly and implants, because of the need for surgery and stitches, don't satisfy that desire.

HUMAN FASCIA (NOT AVAILABLE IN THE UK)

A medical term used to describe the thick sheets of connective tissue that line muscles, fascia has been used safely as a surgical implant for years. Recently, *Fascian* – an injectable particulate form of human fascia that is derived from human cadavers – has become available. With *Fascian*, freeze-dried particles of this connective tissue are combined with a local anaesthetic to create a dense suspension, and that is then implanted into the trouble spots. Due to its origins, some patients are concerned about the risk of disease transmission, but this risk is minimal thanks to the careful screening process that it undergoes. Finally, fascia doesn't seem to last longer than collagen.

SYNTHETIC FILLERS

SILICONE

Silicone is considered to be the black sheep of filler materials, a judgement that is not entirely unfair considering its history of misuse. The biggest complaint about silicone has revolved around its tendency to migrate from its intended location as well as the many impure varieties of silicone that were on the market.

The introduction of *Silikon 1000*, a silicone product that is approved in America for the treatment of certain ophthalmologic conditions, has brought renewed interest in the area of silicone fillers. Some doctors are using *Silikon 1000* as an off-label cosmetic filler. It is not yet approved or available in the UK, but the manufacturer is in the process of implementing the trials necessary for approval for cosmetic use.

If done properly the results with silicone can be excellent, but there are several crucial variables that determine a positive outcome. First, silicone must be injected slowly, with tiny droplets injected in the wrinkle at intervals separated by at least a month, so deep wrinkles can take six months to a year to get fully corrected. Like with other procedures that are classified as permanent, it's important to remember that nothing will keep further wrinkles from showing up. The bottom line is: sooner or later, you'll need to return for a little fine-tuning.

ARTECOLL

A combination of bovine collagen with polymethylmethacrylate, a plexiglas-type sphere that can be injected into deep lines in the face and scars, *Artecoll* has been used in Canada, Europe, Mexico and South America since 1993.

The collagen portion of *Artecoll* eventually disappears, while the sphere remains permanently. Some patients have seen great results with this filler, particularly in the treatment of wrinkles, but others have reported adverse reactions to the sphere, such as the development of lumps in the skin. It's also been noted that *Artecoll* can deliver a bumpy effect to the lips. As *Artecoll* is mixed with bovine collagen, a skin test is required. The injection is administered similarly to collagen, except that some doctors like to tape the treated area for at least two days after the procedure so that the filler is able to settle into place.

My opinion on *Artecoll* is that if a patient is going to use a synthetic substance, it's wiser to use a purely synthetic filler, such as silicone.

IMPLANTS

When filler implants were introduced almost thirty years ago they brought with them great hope in being an answer to the ravages of time. In recent years, however, the initial excitement surrounding filler implants has definitely waned. High on the list of complaints is the tendency of implants to lose their original shape – they can get hard, contract and even protrude from their original location. It is also difficult to achieve the right fit because, unlike injectable fillers, implants are linear and need to conform to a certain shape. Studies are also beginning to show that implants can't be considered permanent. Ageing, as we all know, is a continuous process so what constitutes a major improvement today will be less of one in a year's time. Also, even though implants smooth certain creases really well, such as the nasolabial folds, they don't correct them entirely, making it necessary to have another filler injected over it for a complete correction.

Finally, in my experience I've found that patients want to improve their facial flaws quickly and effortlessly and implants, because of the need for surgery and stitches, don't satisfy that desire.

ALL ABROAD

The following list contains many filler substances that are available in various parts of the world. Unfortunately not all of these have been put through a cautious evaluation process that requires an observation period of at least one year. In my opinion the *Zyderm/Zyplast* bovine collagen formulations, the soon to be *Cosmoderm/Cosmoplast* human derived collagen formulations, as well as the *Restylane* and *Hylaform* family of products provide at this point in time our safest treatment options.

AcHyal
Arteplast
Biocell Ultravital
Bioplastique
DermaLive
DermaDeep
Dermaplant
Endoplast-50
Evolution
Fat Autografting
Formacrill
Human Placental Collagen
Hyal-System

Hylan Rofilan Gel
Kopolymer
Meta-Crill
New-Fill
Permacol
Plasmagel
PMS 350
Profill
Resoplast
Reviderm Intra
Adatosil 5000
Silikon 1000
Surgisis

I think it's clear that collagen, which for years has been the gold standard of filler materials, is being challenged by some pretty serious competition, primarily from the *Restylane* group of materials. In fact, I think that of all the fillers that are currently available, *Restylane* is the one that is really going to shine in the years to come. Not only is it immensely versatile, both in its ability to restore that youthful volume to the face and eliminate those less-than-youthful lines and wrinkles, but it also lasts an incredibly long time and doesn't require a time-consuming skin test. That is a magical combination that I'm certain will leave patients happily and beautifully satisfied. Aside from a permanent antidote to ageing, one couldn't ask for much more.

CHAPTER SIX
RADIANCE REVEALED

What is it about young and healthy skin that elicits a steady stream of compliments? An absence of lines and wrinkles might seem like the obvious answer but actually, that doesn't paint the full picture. It turns out that radiance, which is hard to define but desired by everyone, is what signals to the world that all is well with your skin.

So what is radiance? This nebulous expression is often used to describe those on the brink of a life-changing event – expectant mothers and blushing brides are often at the receiving end of this compliment. Without a doubt, radiance is a term ripe with connotations of happiness, health and vitality. In a medical sense, a look of radiance can be attributed to a variety of elements. For starters, radiant skin is evenly pigmented, its texture is dewy and smooth and the pores are so tiny that they might as well be invisible. The colour of the skin, too, is alive and bright. Put it all together and the end result is the kind of skin that looks beautiful even without a drop of make-up.

By now you're probably thinking that this dream skin is impossible to obtain and clearly only babies and Hollywood starlets can claim it as their own. There is a certain element of truth to that statement since what comprises radiant skin – abundant collagen and elastin, minimal, if any, sun damage and a rapid cell turnover, to name just a few – comes naturally to young people. Over time, however, these elements start to crumble. Even someone who has only just turned thirty can have skin that doesn't replenish itself as quickly as it did just a few years before, resulting in an accumulation of dead skin cells that contribute to how your skin reflects light. Throw in the lines and multiple brown spots that are usually the result of too much sun exposure and it's easy to see why you now possess a dull complexion of your very own.

Now for some good news. There are a multitude of cosmetic resurfacing procedures today that will help you undo most, if not all, of this damage and ultimately reward you with a smooth and glowing complexion. Much like every other goal related to obtaining flawless skin, being satisfied with your result goes hand in hand with an effective at-home skin care regimen. In an earlier chapter I explained how products containing alpha and beta hydroxy acids and retinol, to name just a few ingredients, are crucial because of their ability to thoroughly exfoliate the skin and possibly stir collagen production, in turn ensuring that your complexion remains as smooth and even as possible. But as impactful as these ingredients are in maintaining skin health and reversing some of that past damage, even they have their limitations. Need another solution? Enter the resurfacing treatment.

WHAT IS SKIN RESURFACING?

Just as the name implies, resurfacing treatments rid you of a mottled complexion and replace it with a much improved version of itself. This is accomplished in different ways and to varying degrees, but this much is true: if you don't like what Father Time has done to your skin, then by all means use a resurfacing treatment to improve on his work.

In this chapter I will be reviewing a range of procedures that are unsurpassed for attaining radiant skin. Some of these procedures, like light acid peels, rid the upper layer of the skin (*stratum corneum*) of accumulated dead skin cells and can be found at some spas as well as at the dermatologist's office. At the other end of the spectrum are the more invasive procedures, such as deep peels, dermabrasion and certain lasers that actually penetrate past the *stratum corneum* and into the living tissues of the skin. Once there, the all-important collagen is stimulated and most pigmentation problems are taken care of. This level of resurfacing should only be entrusted to a doctor in a medical setting. The deeper the treatment, the greater the result and, accordingly, the longer the recuperation.

Nestled comfortably between these two extremes are a medley of treatments that deliver a significant enough change with a tolerable amount of discomfort. Certain types of lasers (including the new, non-burning lasers) fall into this category, as do some chemical peels. Completing this group are microdermabrasion treatments.

Whatever your mission – from eradicating those unpleasant reminders of your suntanning years to getting the radiant complexion you've always longed for – I'm pretty certain that you'll find answers here. The all-important question, of course, is which of these treatments is the appropriate one for you and this chapter – and your doctor – will help you decide.

CHEMICAL PEELS

Chemical peels help improve a litany of skin conditions, such as acne, melasma, uneven skin texture, brown spots, hyperpigmentation and wrinkling. The classifications of peeling are typically ranked as very superficial, superficial, medium and deep and once the doctor has assessed the condition of the skin, it is decided which of these four depths of peeling would be the most helpful. The lower intensity peels tend to be very popular, particularly at spas and skin clinics, while medium and deep peels have declined in popularity due in large part to the introduction of new laser procedures. Lasers can often yield the same if not a better result than deep peeling, with significantly less recovery time.

WHAT IS IN A PEEL?

A lot of the same ingredients that are so impactful for at-home skin care are used in much higher concentrations in professional peels. They include the following:

Glycolic acid

The most common ingredient in chemical peels is glycolic acid, one of the star members of the alpha hydroxy group. Like I explained in an earlier chapter, AHAs are derived from naturally occurring compounds, in this case sugar cane, and they work by inducing exfoliation and speeding the cell cycle. The typical concentration of a glycolic acid product tends to be no higher than 10%, while for a peel the concentration can climb up to 70%.

Salicylic acid

As the lone member of the beta hydroxy group, salicylic acid is unrivaled in how well it treats acne-prone skin. For home use, most products feature an average of 2% salicylic acid, while in a peel a typical concentration is 20–30%.

Other peeling agents

Concluding the most utilised peeling ingredients are resorcinol, a phenol derivative that can be used for an in-office peel either on its own, or as a key component of the popular *Jessner's Solution* peel. This popular peel combines a hotchpotch of exfoliating ingredients, including resorcinol, salicylic and lactic acid (also an AHA), and was developed by a dermatologist who sought to reduce the concentration and toxicity of each of the individual ingredients while increasing efficacy. Another benefit of Jessner's Solution is that it can be layered under other peels for even more dramatic improvement.

Usually reserved for superficial and medium depth peels is trichloroacetic acid (TCA). If done repeatedly, a low concentration (usually 10–15%) TCA peel can kill fine wrinkles and leave the skin with a smooth finish. Once the intensity is increased to the standard 35–40% it is able to delve deeper, but with a higher risk of scarring and hyperpigmentation.

The most invasive peel is done with phenol and it can dramatically improve the complexion. It brings myriad disadvantages, however, and like I mentioned earlier, lasers have pretty much taken over where deep peels left off.

Like with every other resurfacing technique mentioned here, I insist that you entrust your face to only the most experienced doctor. So many variables can affect the outcome of a chemical peel, most of which aren't readily apparent. In other words, in the hands of different doctors the same ingredient will deliver a different outcome.

The most basic factor is the type of acid that is used and in what percentage, and in some cases, the pH level. The higher the pH, the more basic the solution; the lower the pH, the more acidic. Other considerations are the technique used in applying the solution. Is it being painted on lightly or rubbed in? How long is it being kept on the skin? How does the doctor prepare the skin prior to the peel? What skin care regime is the patient following? Does it include a regime with highly active ingredients, like *Retin-A*? What kind of skin does the patient have? Is she an Italian woman with thick, oily skin? Or is she a blonde who's had a facelift and has the thinned skin to show for it? The attention paid to these variables is monumental in determining a successful outcome.

Just like the face, the hands, neck and chest are often exposed to the sun and receive their fair share of damage. But unlike the face, which responds extremely well to stronger peels thanks to the rich supply of oil glands there, other areas of the body can't be peeled as deeply without risking scars.

VERY SUPERFICIAL PEELS

Just about everybody can benefit from a very superficial peel, from younger patients with minimal imperfections to older patients who haven't exposed their skin to a lot of sun. The number one benefit of a very superficial peel is its effectiveness at removing the dead skin cells that stubbornly cling to the skin's outer layer, the *stratum corneum*, in the process yielding skin that is smoother in texture and more evenly pigmented. Those with acne can see great improvement, such as in the cleansing of blocked pores and the fading of any leftover dark marks. A patient can also expect the removal of freckles, certain types of melasma and *solar lentigos* (sun spots). Fine wrinkles can be improved considerably, but it does very little for deeper lines. After several treatments, the repetitive peeling action, or exfoliation, can stimulate growth of the epidermis and even lead to regeneration of collagen.

A bit of patience always comes in handy, and it will be put to good use in this instance. Basically, when the peeling is this superficial, it's unrealistic to expect a whole new you after just one treatment. It usually takes at least four peels, spaced approximately two weeks apart, before you can begin to see an improvement.

Suggested peels

⋯⟩ glycolic acid at 30–50% (depending on the pH factor)

⋯⟩ *Jessner's Solution*

⋯⟩ TCA (10–15%)

Recuperation

None. You might be a little pink but nothing that a touch of make-up can't disguise.

Suggested frequency

···} Initially: every three to four weeks
···} Maintenance: every two months

SUPERFICIAL PEELS

Slightly stronger than the level before it, superficial peels penetrate deeper into the epidermis, and are ideal for those with even more sun damage and other texture imperfections.

Suggested peels

···} glycolic acid at 50–70% (depends on the pH factor)
···} resorcinol at 40–50%
···} TCA at 20%

Recuperation

Similar to a very superficial peel, but with additional peeling and flaking of the skin. These effects can last up to a week and in some cases resemble a light sunburn.

Suggested frequency

···} Initially: every ten to fourteen days
···} Maintenance: every four weeks

MEDIUM PEELS

Now we're getting somewhere! Medium-depth peels go past the epidermis and affect the upper portion of the dermis, which is where the blood vessels and the collagen reside. This process of inflaming the skin helps to produce new collagen. Essentially, any time collagen is manipulated it results in a firming action and, further down the road, an increase in natural collagen.

This level of peeling is great for someone with moderate wrinkling and acne. Deep lines will be softened, although not entirely eliminated, while pretty much all brown spots will be erased.

One caveat is that medium-depth peels are generally only appropriate for skin types I to III, as classified by the Fitzpatrick Skin Type system of classifying skin tones. (Refer to *Chapter Two: What Ages Us?* for more information on these classifications.) Darker skin tones, such as those that fall within the range of types IV to VI, can benefit from a medium peel, but if done improperly there is a greater risk of developing post-inflammatory hyperpigmentation.

Suggested peels

→ glycolic acid at 70% (depends on the pH factor)
→ TCA at 35%
→ *Augmented TCA Plus*: glycolic acid at 70% plus TCA at 35%
→ *Carbon Dioxide Flush* plus TCA at 35%

Recuperation

Expect to look pretty bad for the first ten days following a medium-depth peel. On days one and two the skin appears slightly pink. On days three and four, the skin darkens. By day five the skin begins to peel off. Finally, by day ten the peeling should be completed and you'll be able to flaunt your newly rejuvenated self.

Suggested frequency

Once a year

DEEP PEELS

Deep peels are turning into the endangered species of the resurfacing world and anyone familiar with how it works will understand why. This level of peeling is done with phenol, an acid that has the ability to penetrate down to the deepest levels of the skin. For the procedure, the patient is sedated, hooked up to a cardiac monitor and his or her vital signs are repeatedly checked for irregularities. The recuperation time is also lengthy – the skin is raw for two or three weeks with the skin remaining pink for two to three months. Other risks include the possible loss of pigmentation, called hypopigmentation, resulting in the face being much lighter than the neck and body.

On the upside, since the peel is penetrating the skin more deeply, it produces long-lasting and extremely dramatic improvement. By reaching deep into the collagen layer, the skin is able to regenerate more of it. The ideal patient would be one with severe sun damage, such as cross-hatched lines on the cheeks and leathery skin.

Suggested peel

phenol peel

Recuperation

There's no elegant way to word this. After a deep peel the skin is in pretty bad shape for two weeks, and pink for months afterwards.

Suggested frequency

Once in a lifetime

LASER
(Light Amplification by the Stimulated Emission of Radiation)

When the buzz on lasers as an anti-ageing tool first started percolating in the early 1990s, people didn't know what to make of it. To most people, lasers were symbols of the kind of high-tech wizardry associated with the characters in *Star Wars*. Faster than the speed of light, however, lasers went from being a novel idea of the future to a much improved alternative to the cosmetic procedures that already existed.

Almost five years later, laser technology has evolved into a mighty presence for cosmetic improvement. In the past, lasers were limited to the treatment of certain cosmetic conditions such as birth marks that affected only a small group of people.

That all changed with the introduction of the carbon dioxide (CO_2) laser, the first of its kind to actually resurface the skin. Before the CO_2 laser, the only other procedure that could regenerate the superficial and deep layers of skin was a deep phenol peel or dermabrasion. Not long after, it seemed like a new cosmetic laser was being introduced on a daily basis. This innovation radically improved the success rates of treating certain flaws, such as redness and brown spots on the hands and chest.

A lot of my patients tell me that they're afraid of lasers – usually because they assume that there's only one type of (scary) laser – but I reassure them that 'lasers' is just an umbrella term that encompasses different types of lasers. I liken it to how aeroplanes and cars are different forms of transport with similar engineering characteristics.

Lasers work by aiming a beam of amplified light at the skin and when that beam hits the skin, it is attracted to certain components. For example, a laser for brown spots is attracted to melanin, or pigment, and a vascular laser is attracted to the red blood vessels. Since the subject of lasers is vast enough to fill an entire book, we will limit our discussion to the cosmetic lasers that are indispensable for bringing out your beauty.

WHAT ARE LASERS USED FOR?

⟶ Port wine stains and birthmarks

⟶ Wrinkles and lines

⟶ Superficial brown spots

⟶ Deep-pigmented spots

⟶ Scars and stretch marks

⟶ Removing broken blood vessels

⟶ Warts

⟶ Hair removal

⟶ Tattoo removal

ABLATIVE LASERS

The term 'ablative' refers to the act of cutting into the skin. An ablative laser, therefore, is cutting through the skin. (I know it's hard to imagine this since there's not a scalpel in sight!)

Carbon dioxide (CO_2) laser

Almost a decade ago, those people who were contemplating 'getting a little something done' were drawn to lasers and the wrinkle busting and overall skin rejuvenation results that they promised. At the time, the carbon dioxide (CO_2) resurfacing laser, which is still around today, was being touted as a one-stop solution for these conditions, especially severely sun-damaged skin. This laser delivers results comparable to those from a deep phenol peel, minus the health risks. It is also one example of the ablative (or burning) lasers that work by heating the surface of the skin in order to penetrate into the deepest layers. In the case of the CO_2 laser, an amplified wavelength of light is directed at the skin and it is immediately attracted to the water in the skin. Once there, the water absorbs the light, in the process removing years of sun spots, wrinkles and other remnants of accumulated damage. The patient's skin is red and swollen immediately following the treatment, with full recovery coming slowly after several weeks, once new skin has grown in.

If this process sounds serious, that's because it is very serious – a fact that at that time wasn't emphasised nearly enough. Not only is the recovery long and often painful, but it carries serious side effects, such as loss of pigment and scarring. Also, people mistakenly thought that they would never get another wrinkle, which is a nice wish but as we all know definitely untrue. Other patients underestimate the power of this laser and request to treat their few lines with it. For those patients, I reply that this approach is like using a canon to kill a fly.

I think that while CO_2 lasers are great for certain people, they were initially overused. Someone with a few lines doesn't need to be resurfaced. Often, a filler like collagen could be injected instead and successfully alleviate the problem. It's also not for someone with dynamic wrinkles around the eyes. *Botox* is better suited for those types of wrinkles that will only come back. As with any other procedure, the potential use of a CO_2 laser has to be determined on a person by person basis. It's not a magic wand.

Recuperation
Two weeks of no make-up, with the skin remaining pink for two to three months.

Suggested frequency
One or twice in a lifetime

Erbium:YAG Laser
Less dramatic in effect than the CO_2 laser, but nonetheless very effective at improving wrinkles, the *Erbium:YAG* was, and still is today, a moderate alternative to the CO_2 laser. The skin doesn't heat as much with this laser but you also don't get as deep and dramatic a result. It's great for people with mild to moderate sun damage. Again, the Erbium is comparable to a medium-depth peel.

Recuperation
It'll be a week before you can wear make-up, accompanied by a month of redness.

Suggested frequency
Once every five years, if necessary.

PIGMENT LASERS
If someone can easily play 'connect the dots' with the brown spots on your hands, face, shoulders and chest, then you're a great candidate for a treatment with a pigment laser. These spots, typically referred to as 'liver spots', are caused by the irregular melanin production brought on by – what else? – the sun. The specific pigment in the laser acts as a magnet, drawing the light only to the pigment while sparing the surrounding skin.

Common pigment lasers
⋯⋯> *Q-switched ruby*
⋯⋯> *Q-switched alexandrite*
⋯⋯> *Q-switched Nd:YAG*
⋯⋯> *Aura*

Recuperation

Immediately after the treatment, the skin will be red and scabs will start to form. In about a week the facial skin will be sufficiently healed to wear make-up. The hands take about two weeks to heal, the arms three weeks and the legs almost a month. All areas will have some redness for several months afterwards.

Suggested frequency

One session is usually sufficient to remove all visible spotting. But remember, inadequate sun protection will deliver a multitude of new spots.

VASCULAR LASERS

A certain amount of rosiness is always desirable, but not when it's in the form of severe redness on the face, most prominently on the cheeks and around the corners of the nose. This is usually a direct result of dilated or broken blood vessels. Rosacea, a chronic condition that brings about a lot of involuntary blushing, also sees a great benefit with such lasers.

Finally, most types of red birthmarks can quickly be eradicated with this treatment. In this instance, the laser targets the haemoglobin (red pigment in the bloodstream), that lies within the vessels.

Common vascular lasers

...⟩ *VersaPulse*

...⟩ *Aura*

...⟩ *Vbeam*

Recuperation

The skin bounces back almost immediately afterwards.

Suggested frequency

As needed

NON-ABLATIVE (NON-BURNING) LASER RESURFACING

One of the miracles of non-surgical cosmetic treatments, non-ablative laser resurfacing treatments are the perfect solution for those who want to improve their complexions at their own pace. The opposite of ablative lasers, non-ablative treatments work by rejuvenating the skin without removing skin and creating a wound that needs time to heal.

Not surprisingly, one session of a non-ablative treatment won't deliver the same dramatic result as a CO_2. Actually, a series of four to six treatments is required before the patient can see a change. On the upside, the recuperation time is nil.

Common non-ablative lasers

....⟫ *CoolTouch*

....⟫ *SmoothBeam*

....⟫ *N-Lite*

....⟫ *Aura* and *Lyra* laser combination

Recuperation

None whatsoever. You can hop on the exam table and hop right off.

Suggested frequency

Four to six treatments required

INTENSE PULSED LIGHT (IPL)

It's usually mentioned in the same breath as laser treatments, but unlike lasers, which amplify one wavelength of light, this treatment uses a multitude of wavelengths depending on the desired results. And since the energy is not as high and more diffuse, it's not as potent. The ideal conditions for this treatment are hyperpigmentation, freckles, ruddiness, broken blood vessels, early sunspots, large pores, fine lines and lax skin.

Common IPL treatments

....⟫ *IPL Facial*

....⟫ *FotoFacial*

....⟫ *PhotoFacial*

....⟫ *Photorejuvenation*

....⟫ *EpiFacial*

Recuperation

This is a true 'lunchtime' procedure, with no recuperation time whatsoever.

Suggested frequency

Once a month for four months.

COBLATION (ELECTROSURGICAL COLD ABLATION)

Coblation delivers saline to the skin through which a cool electric current is passed. A subsequent reaction specifically heats and vaporises the top layer of skin. Known as *Visage*, it is very effective for mild to moderate wrinkles and sun damage in people with all skin types.

Recuperation

The skin will be tender for five to seven days and overall redness will subside in a month.

Suggested frequency

Once every five years, if necessary.

MECHANICAL EXFOLIATION

Dermabrasion

Dermabrasion is still popular with the doctors who are experienced in it. This is key, since this procedure is truly an inexact science. A rapidly rotating wheel studded with diamond particles deeply abrades the skin and causes the skin to bleed and crust. When done correctly, though, the results are fantastic.

Recuperation

It'll be a week to ten days before you can wear make-up, and several months before the redness subsides.

Suggested frequency

Can be repeated at intervals no greater than every year or two.

Microdermabrasion

There are certain people who adore the idea of scrubbing away all imperfections, and these folks will probably love microdermabrasion. This treatment, which is helpful for improving skin texture, unblocking pores, removing excess oil and possibly reducing wrinkles, works in the following way. As the small microdermabrasion machine bombards the skin with thousands of sterilised aluminium oxide crystals, a vacuum suction removes these particles along with the dislodged skin. The force at which the particles are propelled and the speed at which the device is passed over the skin determine the depth of the treatment. There is a small risk of experiencing certain side effects, such as bleeding, infection, and hyperpigmentation, but overall I think that microdermabrasion can be useful and safe if done by a properly trained doctor. It can also be overused, so I'd advise that it be done no more than twelve to twenty times in a year.

The most common particle is the aluminium oxide crystal, but since the introduction of microdermabrasion just a few years ago, other particles, like salt crystals, are making headlines. There are also more microdermabrasion treatments on the market than there are wrinkles on the face, but essentially they all perform the same function. As a side note, microdermabrasion is equivalent to having a light acid peel.

Common microdermabrasion treatments

···⟩ Dermapeel

···⟩ Power peel

···⟩ Parisian peel

···⟩ Diamond peel

···⟩ Silk peel

Recuperation

Aside from minor pinkness, there are no other adverse effects.

Suggested frequency

No more than twelve to twenty times a year.

There are many ways to get to your desired end point and deciding which route to take should be a joint decision between yourself and your doctor. And, at the risk of sounding like a very broken record, I must stress how important it is to stay out of the sun. Why undergo another procedure when a few simple precautionary steps can keep you beautiful for a long, long time? Point taken? Good.

CHAPTER SEVEN
BEFORE & AFTER

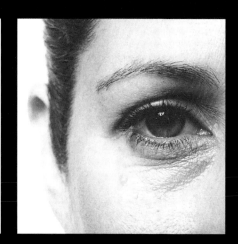

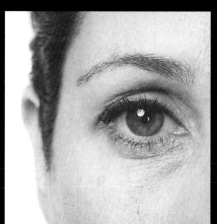

It's been said that a picture paints a thousand words, and this is never truer than when the topic is the transformative powers of today's non-surgical cosmetic procedures. One of my missions in this book has been to provide you with the basic facts regarding these procedures, and while I hope I've done that, I understand that words can only say so much. Without a doubt, it's one thing for you to read all about these new techniques and quite another to actually see them put to the test. And have we put them to the test! Read on as Andrea, Linda, Maija and Brenda, our four female volunteers – who range in age from 39 to 54 – candidly describe the specific ways that ageing is affecting their looks. Their motivations for submitting their

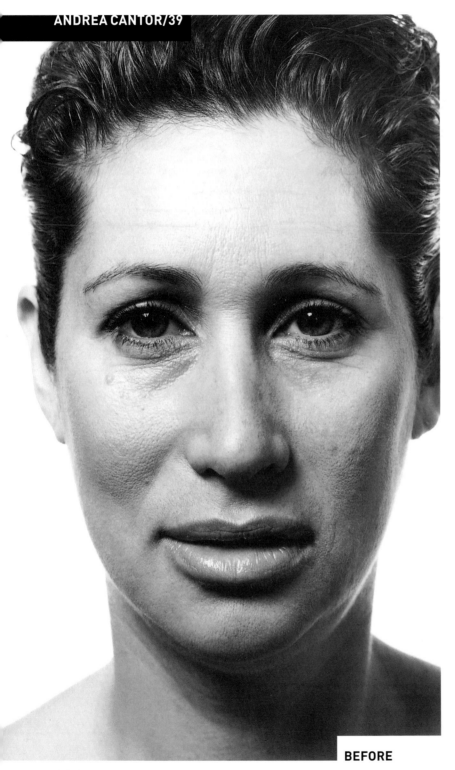

ANDREA CANTOR/39

BEFORE

DR BRANDT'S VIEW

'Talk about a busy life. In the midst of raising three young daughters with her husband and co-running a successful publicity firm in Westchester, New York, Andrea Cantor stopped moving long enough one day to realise that the big 4-0 was just around the corner. It didn't matter when friends assured her that she looked very youthful (which she did and does). She was adamant to greet this milestone of a birthday with a little beautification.

'For someone like Andrea, who had never had a cosmetic procedure and who didn't need plastic surgery yet, *Botox* was truly the way to go. I studied her face and made a few determinations. First, like a lot of women her age, Andrea was starting to have a lot of loose tissue under eyes and lines around them. She also had a bulge under her eyes that she wasn't even aware of! This area is commonly mistaken for an accumulation of fat when in fact it's an overworked muscle that can benefit from *Botox*. By injecting that bulge I was able to clean up her lower eyelid area without a need for surgery. Finally, I noted that Andrea was starting to get some jowl formation and her jawline was starting to lose definition, so despite her initial shock, we decided to give her a little *Botox* there, too.

'The forehead area has some lines as well, which I treated, but I intentionally didn't completely erase them, because to take that approach would have lowered her brows. This combination of moderately treating her forehead and brows allowed her eyes to open up wide and make her look very alert, which is exactly what she wanted. I think Andrea will be welcoming her fortieth birthday beautifully!'

Homecare prescription

⋯⟩ *v-zone neck cream* will maintain firmness and elasticity in the neck area as well as smooth skin texture.
⋯⟩ *lineless eye cream* to reduce puffiness and dark circles, promote firmness and smooth signs of ageing.

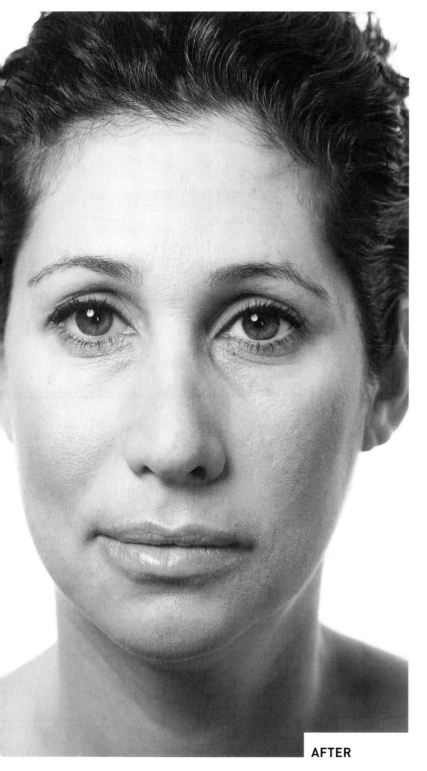

AFTER

ANDREA'S VIEW

'I am about to turn forty – ouch! – and I told my husband that for my birthday I wanted a little lift and softness around my eyes, mainly so that I wouldn't always look so tired. I also said I'd consider a tummy tuck, but I would never really go through with it and I figured the cosmetic treatment would be more realistic. I guess I was looking for the instant shot (no pun intended!) of gratification. For almost a year now, I had been contemplating having *Botox* and the desire has only grown stronger. In fact, I had just started to look into making an appointment with a dermatologist when this opportunity arose.

'I was very excited about the procedure, not really nervous at all, and I was particularly looking forward to meeting the infamous Dr Brandt. I'd heard and read so much about him. He has so much experience with *Botox* and if anyone was qualified to shoot me up, I felt that he was definitely the one. My only fear was that my facial expressions would look forced. Plastic surgery never truly entered my mind, both because I've seen a lot of bad plastic surgery and I thought I was too young for that, anyway. Maybe my feelings will change as I get older, but I find the idea of going under the knife to be very unnerving. I'm hoping that genetics, a good skin care regime and proper sun protection will go a long way.

'On the day of the treatment, I opted to have the numbing cream applied to my face for approximately thirty minutes beforehand. I'm sure that helped, because the procedure didn't really hurt much with the exception of the area between my brows. The nurse had warned me that since that particular area has the thickest muscle it might feel a bit uncomfortable. The only other slightly freaky part was when he injected my lower eyelid. I was not expecting that – I didn't even know that that area needed treating – and it was frightening to see a needle coming towards my eye!

'At one point, Dr Brandt said that he was going to treat my neck and I thought he was joking. But sure enough, he started studying that area and before long he was asking me to make clenching motions. The injections there were absolutely painless – it was hard to believe he was truly treating my neck.

'Overall, I am quite pleased with the results since they are very subtle and natural looking. The areas around my eyes look softer, but I am not quite sure that I see a difference in the vertical lines by my brows. I would most definitely go back for more treatments. It was a great experience and I would tell others that it's a fast, mostly painless way to get an instant boost. And, by the way, my husband thinks I look wonderful.'

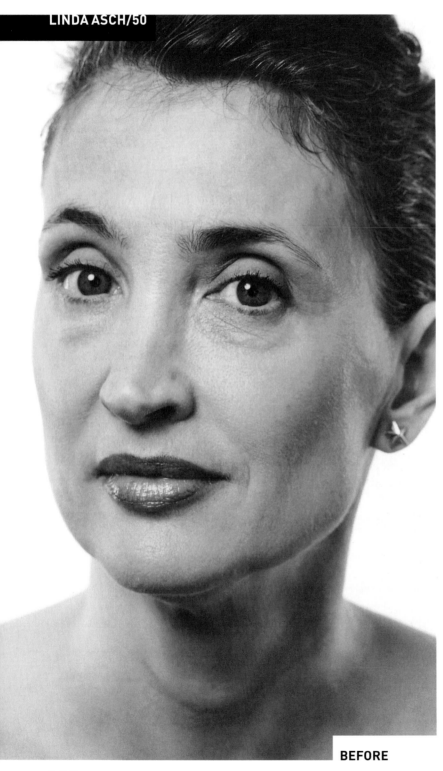

LINDA ASCH/50

DR BRANDT'S VIEW

'There are many reasons why people decide to enhance their appearance and in the case of Linda Asch, it truly had a higher meaning. Her beloved husband had succumbed to cancer just a few months earlier and during his illness, Linda never had the time, or the inclination, to take a good look in the mirror. In her grief, she even stopped taking yoga classes, which used to bring her such great joy.

'When I met Linda, she told me that she'd had silicone injections in her smile lines, as well as *Botox*, all years earlier. The silicone was still in place but any remnants of the *Botox* were long gone. I was struck by how beautiful her skin was, but nevertheless, as I studied her face, I pinpointed her troubled areas. They included her eyes, which were slightly drooping and the looseness in her neck and the jowls that were beginning to accumulate along her jaw. Luckily for Linda, these are the areas that *Botox* is unrivalled at treating so I used it everywhere: on her neck to eliminate the lines there and create nice definition in her jawline; around her eyes to open them up; on her brows; a dash on the moderately deep lines on her forehead; and even in the chin since she was showing signs of dimpling in that area.

'You'll be the judge, but doesn't Linda look as beautiful on the outside as she is on the inside?'

Homecare prescription

⋯⟩ *c gel* will firm and restore radiance to the skin, reducing free radicals induced by stress.
⋯⟩ *'a' cream night* to rejuvenate the appearance of tired skin, smooth away fine lines and wrinkles as well as stimulate collagen.

BEFORE

128

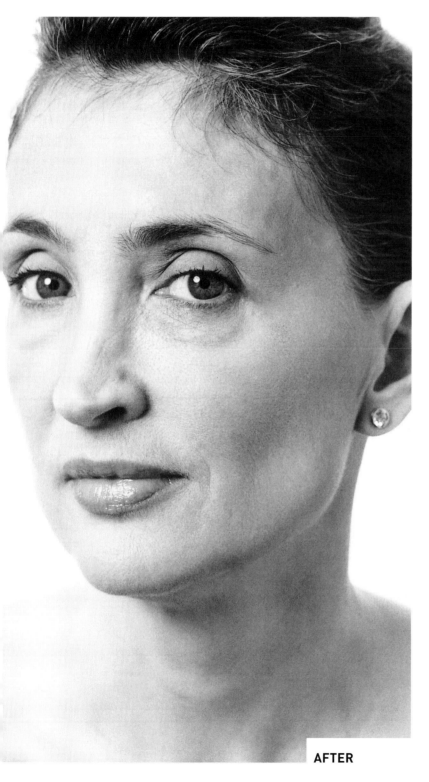

AFTER

LINDA'S VIEW

'Turning fifty years old wasn't such a big deal for me. I've always been very physically active so I was not as much beauty-conscious as I was body-conscious. I spent six months taking care of my husband and there came a point when I couldn't do yoga anymore. Actually, I couldn't really leave the house to follow any kind of normal routine.

'After he passed away, I took the first long look at myself in the mirror and I felt like I had aged. I'd been participating in a bereavement group for a while, and at some point I thought that it would be nice to treat myself to a rejuvenating procedure.

'Four years ago, I had *Botox* on my frown lines and I was looking forward to doing it again. I had once thought that I could grow old gracefully, but now I hope to grow old gracefully with non-surgical procedures! I think it's all a mindset. I think that Jessica Tandy was beautiful. I also loved Gloria Steinman's answer to someone who told her she looked good for being fifty, "This is what fifty looks like". I feel the same way.

'I know that *Botox* isn't really botulism, so I don't really worry about it too much. Dr Brandt's nurse came into the exam room with a bucket of needles but I guess it was all worth it since no one's told me "Oh, you've had *Botox*!" Instead, they comment on how rested I look. After the year I've had, I take that as a great compliment.'

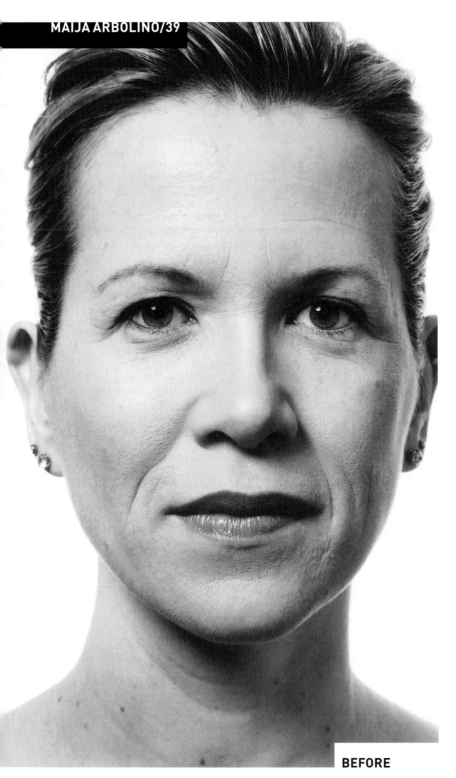

DR BRANDT'S VIEW

'Between her constant travels around the world for her career, and zipping around after her energetic toddler, Maija has been too preoccupied with life to do much more than the basics with her appearance. She is a young woman, but she's already exhibiting a lot of the facial changes that you would see in a fair-skinned person who's had a lot of sun exposure. She needed total face rejuvenation, and using techniques like *Botox*, collagen and *Perlane* allowed me to restore her youthful appearance by filling instead of pulling the skin. A facelift would remove any extra skin in her neck but it would only make her face narrower and do little else for her overall appearance

'I also decide to use *Botox* in her forehead, between the brows, on the neck – basically, everywhere. For her prominent nasolabial creases and marionette lines, I used collagen. I also treated the borders of her lips with collagen, which would eliminate any lipstick bleeding. Lastly, I thought that *Perlane* would be great at building up her cheekbones.

'In my opinion, Maija's 'after' picture could easily be a picture of herself from when she was in her twenties!'

Homecare prescription

⋯⟩ *'c' cream* will address dehydration, discoloration due to sun exposure and minimise fine lines and wrinkles.
⋯⟩ *lightening gel* fades sun and age spots, as well as hyperpigmentation quickly and efficiently.

BEFORE

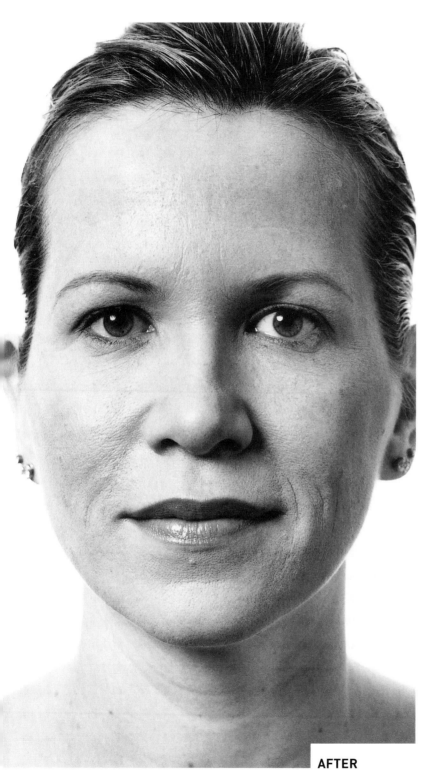

AFTER

MAIJA'S VIEW

'I had a horrifying realisation the other day. Not only was I about to turn forty, but I also look it! All of my life I've always looked younger than my age and ageing somehow snuck up on me. What used to be cute dimples on my cheeks have turned into deep creases. I was also becoming obsessed with my other creases, both around my eyes and on my forehead. And where did this weird "crêpiness" come from? I've seen other women who are my age and their skin looks way better. I'm sure it's from my years of being out in the sun and from thinking that I was indestructible. I've always thought I looked better with a tan – I still think I look better with a tan – but I now believe self-tanning is the only way to go.

'I had been thinking that maybe it was time to get a little something done, but I wanted it to be something that didn't include going under the knife. I've seen some really good facelifts so I know it's possible, but if you can tell you've had a lift, then that's not a good thing. Also, I figured that with surgery you could get a blood clot and die from your facelift. Wouldn't that be a really stupid way to die?

'The possibility of *Botox* was already in my radar. I had been hearing a lot about it and the fact that it was a form of botulism didn't scare me. I like the fact that it's temporary and besides, I hadn't heard about anyone dropping dead from it.

'It was so hectic in his office that day. I had already gotten over my initial apprehension and concerns of what I was going to look like, especially since I've never even had a facial. Finally, Dr Brandt breezes in with these wild glasses on his face, says hello, and starts to scope my face. He was very to the point but also very entertaining. He's like the rock star of the dermatology world. I didn't think the *Botox* was very painful at all and on my neck it was literally painless. On my car ride home, I had to make all of these crazy faces. A few days later, it must have kicked in because I really noticed a difference.

'I was waiting for the results from my two collagen tests so I knew that I had to return for the rest of my treatments. On that second visit, Dr Brandt injected my smile lines and my "commas" around my mouth with collagen and with *Restylane* around my cheekbones. Those injections were less painful than *Botox*.

'I think that I finally look like I've caught up on my sleep. With the results that I got, I would seriously consider doing it all again. I'm already dreading the day that it's all disappeared. I don't want those creases back. My identical twin sister is also carefully watching me and I think she's using me as guinea pig before having anything done to herself. These treatments have also really come in handy at work, particularly when people tell me things that I find ridiculous. I have a better poker face now.'

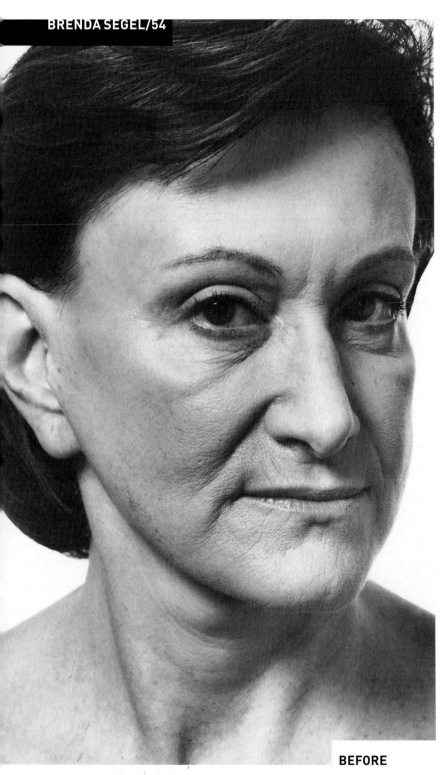

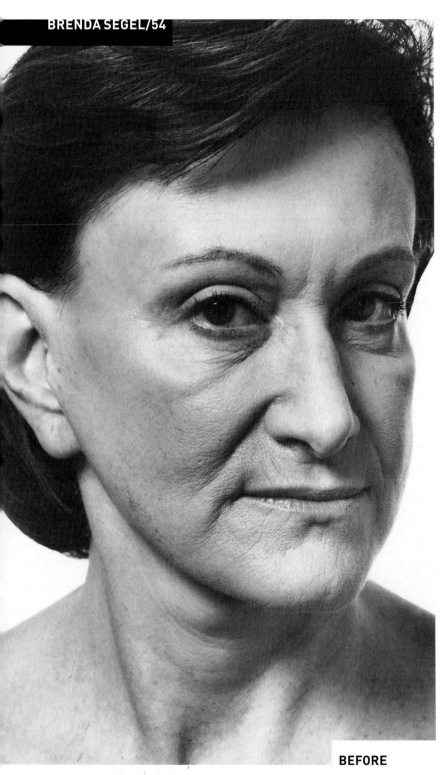

BRENDA SEGEL/54

DR BRANDT'S VIEW

'There's something about significant birthdays that steers people into going through with that nagging desire to have "something done". Brenda grew up hearing her mother's many (well-intentioned) insistences that she have her nose "fixed", a fixation that started when Brenda graduated high school and which went largely unheeded until a monumental birthday, her fortieth, landed her in a plastic surgeon's office for that long-anticipated nose job.

'Almost fifteen years later, the temptation to tinker with her looks surfaced again, and this time Brenda opted to go with *Botox* and collagen injections.

'When I first met Brenda, I noticed that her skin was starting to take on the characteristics usually seen in women in their fifties: her jawline was sagging and her cheeks appeared deflated. She also had a bit of wrinkling around her eyes and on her forehead. For these reasons, I felt that Brenda was a perfect candidate for *Perlane*, the thickest form of *Restylane*, that new hyaluronic acid injectable filler out of Sweden that is generating such media buzz. Brenda was intrigued to hear that I was going to treat her with *Perlane* instead of collagen; she loved the idea that this was the most durable material available today.

'Of course, I also used quite a bit of *Botox* on her, but I didn't concentrate it in one specific area. Thanks to the versatility of *Botox*, I was able to use it throughout her entire face including her neck, on her crow's-feet, under the eyes and on the brows to give her a beautiful lift (a.k.a. The *Botox* Facelift!). I think she looks amazing!'

Homecare prescription

⋯⟩ *lineless cream* to restore a healthy glow to the skin while minimising fine lines and wrinkles.
⋯⟩ *'c' eye cream* to firm the eye contour, maintaining optimal hydration and smoothing signs of ageing.

BEFORE

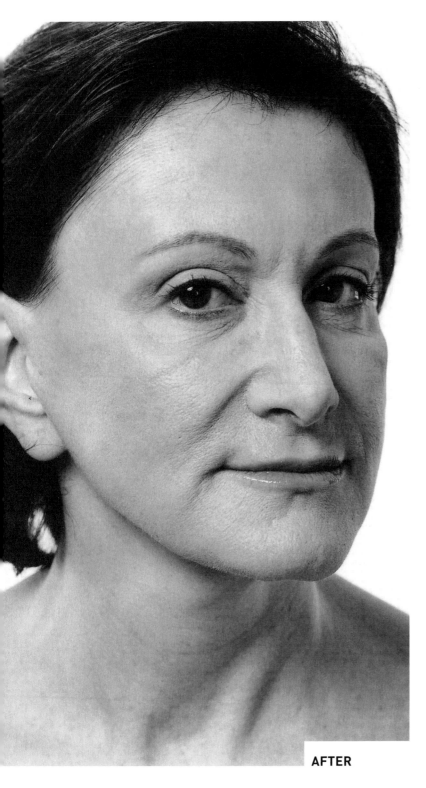

AFTER

BRENDA'S VIEW

'I might not be one of those people who is forever looking in the mirror, but I do feel better if I think I look better, be it through a good haircut, a nice new outfit, or *Botox*. We live in a time when people are living longer. Most of us "baby boomers" don't feel that we are the age that we really are, so we're often shocked when we see pictures of ourselves. It's now possible to improve the picture quite safely, and if it makes you feel better about yourself, why not? Isn't that the whole point?

'I was very excited about meeting Dr Brandt since his reputation is so stellar. I've had both *Botox* and collagen before, by more than one doctor, and I must say that I now realise that technique is everything. While all my previous treatments showed results, none were as striking as those by Dr Brandt. He injected *Botox* not just between the eyes, but above the brows, too. It's like having a brow lift and all of a sudden your eyes are slightly larger and people start telling you how good you look. Also, with him, the *Botox* injections hardly hurt at all – and that was without any numbing cream.

'The *Perlane* was a bit more painful, but tolerable. I was numbed with cream for about twenty minutes before the procedure and when it was time for the big moment, he injected me everywhere! He treated my cheeks, the frown lines from my nose to the corners of my mouth and the fine lines around my lips. Funnily enough, the first time I met Dr Brandt he told me he wanted to do "something about those lips". I was a little nervous, since I fear looking like certain celebrities with overdone lips who shall remain nameless, but I was nonetheless excited to entrust my face to him. There was some stinging and burning afterwards, but the cool gel pads that were placed on my skin did the trick. I had dinner out with a friend an hour later.

'Years ago, my collagen injections had tried to treat my lines that run from the nose to the corners of the mouth and the change was so subtle, it hardly seemed worth it. Having the *Perlane* injected into the cheeks first lifted the skin, so the lines were less prevalent and less heavy. He followed that with injections in the lines and the result was dramatically better. Again, technique was everything.

'The doctor worked quickly and expertly and he always asked me how I was doing. He is delightful and obviously passionate about what he does. He sees this as a labour of love and he is a real artist. The results have more than met my expectations and I would definitely consider doing it again, probably as a touch-up here and there after a few months have passed.'

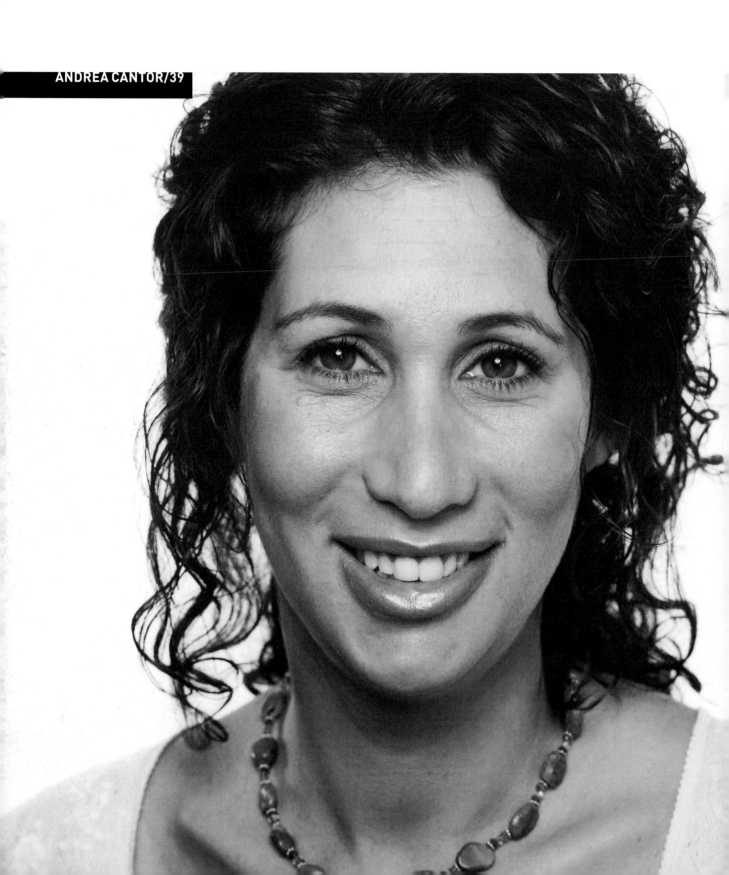

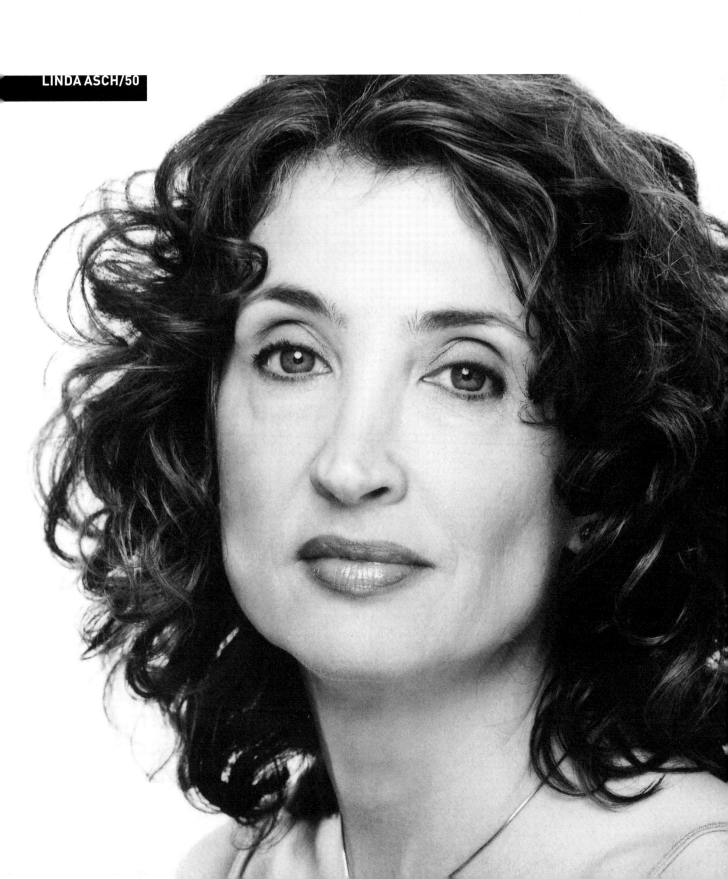

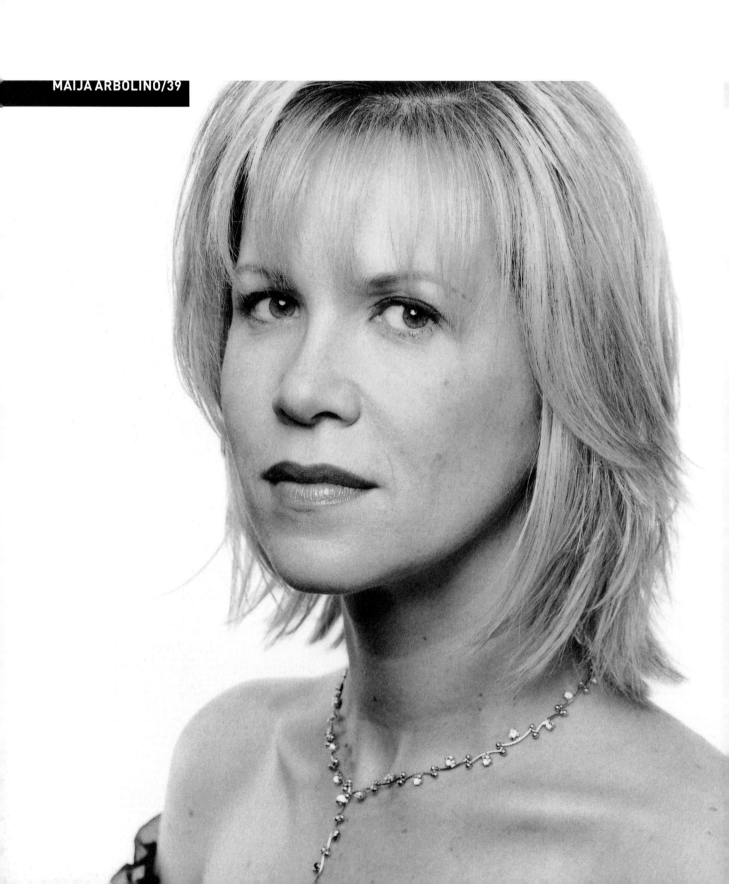

MAIJA ARBOLINO/39

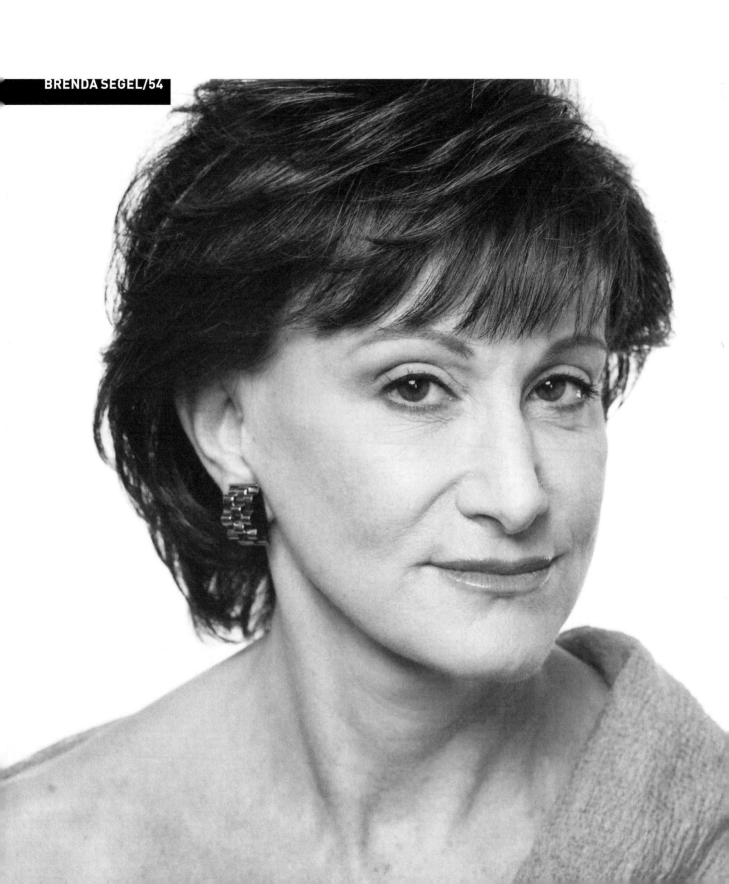

APPENDIX

THE DR. BRANDT SKIN CARE COLLECTION MERGES BOTANICALS, ANTIOXIDANTS AND A MEDLEY OF OTHER ACTIVE, REJUVENATING INGREDIENTS INTO ONE COMPREHENSIVE LINE-UP.

The dr. brandt skin care collection is a healthy lifestyle for mind, body and senses. When it is thought of as a nutritional programme for the skin, the daily diet – its basic bread and butter, so to speak – can be found in the core lineless or poreless products. If your skin category is normal, dry or sensitive, your daily care is in the lineless category. If your skin is combination or oily, you would select a daily diet of products from the poreless category. When your skin is feeling a little under the weather, the active ingredients in the dr. brandt skin care product help your skin regain its sparkle. These products are formulated under dermatological control for maximum safety and efficiency and offer the highest performance without a prescription.

DR. BRANDT SKIN CARE

LINELESS COLLECTION

Antioxidant, anti-wrinkle and anti-ageing prevention and repair is at the heart of Dr Brandt's philosophy. The lineless collection merges sky-high percentages of green tea – the antioxidant superpower known for its skin-saving, anti-inflammatory properties – with grape seed extract, renowned for its protecting, firming, and strengthening power. From the deepest cellular level of the skin up to the surface, the lineless collection smoothes, protects, repairs and adds visible radiance to your skin.

lineless gel cleanser: Green tea, vitamins A and E, and conditioners calm and cleanse in one step.

lineless tone for dry/sensitive skin: An antioxidant toner enriched with witch hazel and chamomile that refreshes and enriches.

lineless cream: Green tea, grape seed extract and botanicals provide anti-ageing benefits in a luxurious cream formula – ideal for normal to dry skin.

lineless gel: Green tea, grape seed extract and botanicals provide anti-ageing benefits in a light weight gel formula – ideal for combination and oily skin.

lineless eye cream: Rich in soothing and firming vitamins, botanicals and green tea for a younger looking eye contour.

lineless soothing mask: A unique mask with green tea and aloe to refresh, revive and renew the complexion.

PORELESS COLLECTION

Formulated for acne-prone skin of all ages, the poreless collection refines enlarged pores, controls excess oil and balances combination complexions. Anti-irritant and lipid soluble salicylic acid is partnered with anti-bacterial tea tree to go deep into the pores, dissolving dirt and oils and clearing breakouts. Calming botanicals and zinc oxide reduce the appearance of redness and the uneven skin tone associated with blemished skin.

poreless cleanser: Formulated with citric extracts to dissolve impurities, oils and debris and leaves you with that ultra-clean sensation.

poreless tone for oily/combination: An invigorating, purifying toner for combination and oily skins.

pore effect: Clarifying cream that combines the power of salicylic acid, anti-bacterial tea tree and stimulating rosemary extract. Soothing lavender calms redness and irritations associated with blemished skin. Used daily, skin becomes visibly clearer with fewer breakouts. Tightens and refines pores and controls excess oils.

poreless moisture: Balancing ultra-sheer moisture formula for oily and combination skin that will not clog pores and is fragrance free. Formulated with soothing lavender and toning white birch to condition skin.

poreless purifying mask: Formulated with kaolin and bentonite clays and tea tree to deep clean, draw out impurities and tighten enlarged pores. Zinc oxide calms redness.